about
CANCER

"An absolutely essential guide for humanity. The little-known wisdom found in this book can help end human suffering across the globe while saving people from the ravages of the failed cancer industry."

— Mike Adams, the "Health Ranger" and
lab science director of CWC Labs

"Ty Bollinger does it again! After the groundbreaking and paradigm-shifting documentary The Truth about Cancer, *Ty's latest book is a comprehensive guide to the cancer epidemic and a holistic solution. Especially intriguing is the information on how sound, light, and electricity are used to boost immune function and heal the body. This book is perfect for those looking to prevent cancer and seeking a natural protocol for treatment."*

— Jack Wolfson, D.O., F.A.C.C.

"Ty Bollinger provides patients, scientists, and health care professionals with an excellent explanation of why our current cancer model is flawed, how cancer can be prevented, and offers a more complete 'menu' of treatment options that are far more favorable on a risk-to-benefit-to-cost ratio when compared to most standard oncology protocols. Use this book as your treasure map to both prevent and reverse cancer. Cancer can be beaten and Ty shows us how."

— Patrick Quillin, Ph.D., R.D., C.N.S., F.A.C.N.,
author of *Beating Cancer with Nutrition*

*"*The Truth about Cancer *is a road map to successfully preventing, treating, and beating cancer with God's medicine chest. In this groundbreaking book, Ty Bollinger sheds light on the plethora of natural ways to promote immunity, fuel the body, and stifle cancer. Read this '*

—Josh A

The
TRUTH
about
CANCER

ALSO BY TY M. BOLLINGER

Cancer: Step Outside the Box

A Guide to Understanding Herbal Medicines and
Surviving the Coming Pharmaceutical Monopoly

Monumental Myths of the Modern Medical Mafia and Mainstream Media

Work with Your Doctor to Diagnose and Cure
27 Ailments with Natural and Safe Methods

TY M. BOLLINGER

The
TRUTH
about
CANCER

WHAT YOU NEED TO KNOW

ABOUT CANCER'S HISTORY,

TREATMENT AND PREVENTION

HAY HOUSE

Carlsbad, California • New York City • London
Sydney • Johannesburg • Vancouver • New Delhi

First published and distributed in the United Kingdom by:
Hay House UK Ltd, Astley House, 33 Notting Hill Gate, London W11 3JQ
Tel: +44 (0)20 3675 2450; Fax: +44 (0)20 3675 2451; www.hayhouse.co.uk

Published and distributed in the United States of America by:
Hay House Inc., PO Box 5100, Carlsbad, CA 92018-5100
Tel: (1) 760 431 7695 or (800) 654 5126
Fax: (1) 760 431 6948 or (800) 650 5115; www.hayhouse.com

Published and distributed in Australia by:
Hay House Australia Ltd, 18/36 Ralph St, Alexandria NSW 2015
Tel: (61) 2 9669 4299; Fax: (61) 2 9669 4144; www.hayhouse.com.au

Published and distributed in the Republic of South Africa by:
Hay House SA (Pty) Ltd, PO Box 990, Witkoppen 2068
info@hayhouse.co.za; www.hayhouse.co.za

Published and distributed in India by:
Hay House Publishers India, Muskaan Complex, Plot No.3, B-2,
Vasant Kunj, New Delhi 110 070
Tel: (91) 11 4176 1620; Fax: (91) 11 4176 1630; www.hayhouse.co.in

Distributed in Canada by:
Raincoast Books, 2440 Viking Way, Richmond, B.C. V6V 1N2
Tel: (1) 604 448 7100; Fax: (1) 604 270 7161; www.raincoast.com

Indexer: Jay Kreider; Cover design: Charles McStravick; Interior design: Alex Head/Draft Lab LLC
Interior photos: Courtesy of the author

The moral rights of the author have been asserted.

The information given in this book should not be treated as a substitute for professional medical
advice; always consult a medical practitioner. Any use of information in this book is at the reader's
discretion and risk. Neither the author nor the publisher can be held responsible for any loss, claim
or damage arising out of the use, or misuse, of the suggestions made, the failure to take medical
advice or for any material on third party websites.

A catalogue record for this book is available from the British Library.

ISBN: 978-1-78180-761-3

Printed and bound in Great Britain by
TJ International Ltd, Padstow, Cornwall

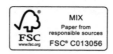

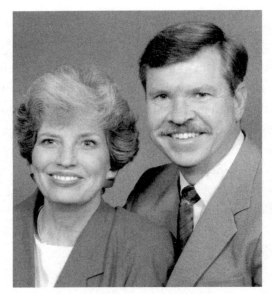

The last picture of Mom and Dad – taken in 1995

This book is dedicated to my mom, Jerry Jean Bollinger-Taylor, and my dad, Charles Graham Bollinger. The best parents I could have ever asked for, and they both loved me unconditionally. I lost both of these amazing people to cancer and its ineffective treatments. In different ways, they were each my hero. When I look back on my life, I can honestly say that I do not have a single bad memory of Mom and Dad. Their smiles were contagious, and so was their zest for life. Now that they are both gone, there are two holes in my heart that will never be filled. But I will see them both again in Heaven. That is my hope.

CONTENTS

FOREWORD

Ty Bollinger is a man on a mission. His powerful message—that cancer is not a death sentence and that anyone anywhere can activate the body's miraculous, God-given healing potential—brings hope to millions around the globe.

The subject of conquering cancer through natural health principles runs deep within my family.

More than a century ago, my great-grandfather Moshe escaped the Russian Army when the then czar was trying to destroy the Jews and immigrated to the United States (his name was changed to Max upon arriving here). He left Russia with nothing, arriving at Staten Island with only the clothes on his back. Somehow, Max became a dental technician and eventually was able to open up his own dental laboratory in Brooklyn.

When he ground down the molds for false teeth and bridges, copious amounts of dust became airborne. He would choke on the dust, and to clear this throat he drank soda. In fact, he drank as many as eight cans each day. After some time, Max complained of severe stomach pain and burning and developed gastritis, followed by ulcers. Despite his symptoms, he wouldn't stop drinking soda. When the ulcers bled, Max went to the hospital, and after a battery of tests he was diagnosed with stomach cancer.

The doctors had nothing to offer him, but somehow my great-grand-father found out about a German doctor named Max Gerson, who treated cancer with a unique diet program. Gerson operated a natural health clinic in Hyde Park, New York, just one and a half hours from New York City, where Max lived. After a short few months on the Gerson protocol, Max became cancer free.

My grandfather became a dentist and my father a naturopathic doctor and chiropractor. I grew up in a home that practiced princi-ples of natural health. It wasn't until I was diagnosed with "incurable" Crohn's disease, and after 69 conventional and natural medicine experts failed to help me, that I realized my calling was to coach others like me to overcome disease. I was able to regain my health only after I met a man who taught me how to eat a real foods diet based on the Bible, proven through history and confirmed by science.

Upon conquering my illnesses, I embarked on a career in natural health, studying sports medicine, naturopathic medicine, and nutri-tion; writing health and wellness publications; and starting multiple nutrition companies. During the early part of my career, my grand-mother Rose was diagnosed with metastatic cancer, and after a surgical procedure to debulk the tumor, she opted against further treatment. She turned to me for help. Based on her uncertain prognosis, I feared she wouldn't survive long enough to attend my upcoming wedding.

I began to research some key natural elements to boost her immune system. I encouraged Grandma Rose to incorporate raw juices and fermented foods into her diet, as well as body therapies for detoxifi-cation. I created nutritional formulations containing combinations of medicinal mushrooms, probiotics, and fermented foods, which she consumed daily. A few months later, she was cancer free. She lived the rest of her life with vim and vigor.

In the summer of 2008, I came face-to-face with the beast we call cancer after an exploratory surgery to correct a suspected hernia revealed a malignancy. When further testing led to a diagnosis of aggressive metastatic cancer that could take my life in a few short months without radical treatment, I took action. Through the potent combination of faith in God my healer and an aggressive nutrition and detoxification program, I became more than a conqueror. I am now eight years removed from the doctor's "death sentence," continuing my crusade to bring health and hope to the world.

I had the privilege of meeting Ty Bollinger years ago, but it wasn't until I participated in his groundbreaking documentary that I had the opportunity to spend time with this true health crusader. Since that time, I have spent countless hours with Ty, and on each visit, it is more and more evident that he truly is a man on a mission.

This book, *The Truth about Cancer*, is a phenomenal reference guide for anyone and everyone who wants to understand cutting-edge protocols to boost nutrition and simultaneously reduce toxins, both of which are critical steps to overcoming cancer. It is a must-read for anyone trying to prevent or conquer cancer.

The Truth about Cancer will open your eyes to a world of options to boost your immune system, reduce inflammation, and help you in the battle for your health and life. This book is your roadmap to greater health and a more abundant life. If you are, or anyone you know and love is, battling the beast called cancer, *The Truth about Cancer* can arm you with powerful health information and, most of all, hope.

If you or a loved one find yourself in a battle with cancer, or you have a family history of the disease and want to ensure a healthy future, I strongly encourage you to carefully explore the natural treatments discussed in this groundbreaking book.

It just may save your health and your life.

Jordan Rubin
Author, *Planet Heal Thyself*
Founder, Ancient Nutrition

INTRODUCTION

A hundred years ago, it was estimated that only 1 in 80 Americans was diagnosed with cancer. According to the World Health Organization, one in two men alive today and one in three women will face a cancer diagnosis.[1]

Most families have been touched by cancer. My family is no exception. Since my wife, Charlene, and I got married in 1995, we have undergone devastating personal losses due to cancer. My dad, Graham Bollinger, was the first casualty. He was diagnosed with stomach cancer on July 1, 1996, and he died on July 25, just 25 days later. He was only 52. Over the course of the next eight years, I lost both of my grandfathers, one grandmother, a cousin, an uncle, and finally my precious mother, Jerry Bollinger-Taylor, to cancer and its ineffective treatments.

During the weeks just before Dad died, I began my "cancer journey." I went to libraries to read books and magazines, since the Internet wasn't all that populated with data back in 1996. Eventually I began to research medical journals, PubMed, the National Library of Medicine, and other reputable sources of information. I began to interview cancer patients who had effectively utilized a natural method to treat their cancer.

My cancer journey continues to this day. Over the past couple of years, I have literally traveled the globe, meeting all kinds of people in the health care world, from practitioners to patients, from North America to Europe to Australia, interviewing them about what treatment protocols are currently being utilized in their area of the world. These interviews, discoveries, and conversations are included in this book.

After doing literally thousands of hours of research over the past 20 years, what I have discovered has truly amazed me. Not only have I learned about the incredible effectiveness of many alternative cancer treatments and the remarkable recoveries of literally thousands of supposedly terminal cancer patients, but I have also learned about the medical industry's suppression of these treatments and persecution of the courageous and innovative medical mavericks who developed these treatments. I have learned about the politics of cancer and the greed of the pharmaceutical companies. I have learned about the war between proponents of conventional and alternative cancer treatments. I am saddened that both Dad and Mom would probably be alive today if knowledge of these alternative cancer treatments had been made available to the public.

Another interesting thing I have learned is that alternative cancer treatments involve much, much more than just taking a quick trip to the local health food store and buying a few bottles of vitamins and minerals. The science behind these treatments is truly remarkable. The specific mechanisms by which certain protocols fight cancer are amazing. As a matter of fact, several alternative cancer treatments have been developed by Nobel Prize winners.

This book contains three parts. Part I lays the foundation for the rest of the book. In it, you will learn about the history of medicine and the politics of cancer treatments. Information on cancer diagnosis, detection, and causes is covered in Part II, while Part III goes into depth on specific cancer treatment protocols that have been proven effective; each chapter in Part III ends with a list of practical takeaways titled "What You Need to Know." If you're facing a cancer diagnosis, you might want to turn straight to Part III and begin learning about these protocols.

In the Bible, we read in Hosea 4:6 that "my people perish for lack of knowledge." One thing I see as I travel across the country and lecture on the subject of cancer is that most people are aware of their "conventional options" for cancer treatment (such as chemotherapy and radiation), but only a small percentage are aware that other "natural options" even exist. The purpose of this book is to educate and empower you with knowledge about these natural options, not to convince or persuade you. I believe in the freedom to choose one's own medical treatment plan, but it's not a real choice if all possible options aren't on the table. Only then can a true choice be made.

This book is for medical practitioners and laypeople alike. It is for cancer patients and non–cancer patients as well. And this book is especially for cancer patients who are currently undergoing, or have already undergone, conventional treatments like chemotherapy, as many of the treatments contained herein can be used in combination with conventional treatments to make them work even better. There are many good physicians who are open to an integrative approach to cancer treatment, and I suggest you find one who can help you design an integrated treatment plan, if that is your desire.

Most people have neither the money nor the time to buy and read the numerous books that have been published on the medical, financial, and political aspects of cancer as well as effective natural and integrative treatment protocols. I am optimistic that this book will serve as a concise yet comprehensive source of information on the subject.

My desire is that other families do not have to suffer loss like my family has suffered. That is the reason I wrote this book. My love for humanity has driven me to devote my life to spreading the truth about cancer to the world. This is my life's mission.

Always remember that cancer is not a death sentence. There is always hope.

Enjoy the book.

—Ty

Part I

The History of Medicine and the Politics of Cancer

CHAPTER 1

HIPPOCRATES, JENNER, AND PASTEUR: MEDICINE'S BEGINNINGS

The body of man has in itself blood, phlegm, yellow bile, and black bile; these make up the nature of the body, and through these he feels pain or enjoys health."

This pithy credo by Hippocrates of Kos (460–circa 370 B.C.), the famous Greek physician who is widely regarded as the "father of Western medicine," was pivotal in the formation of what has come to be known today as modern medicine. It's a belief system that views human health from the perspective of unified wholeness as opposed to a compilation of isolated parts, and it's also the system from which we inherited the concept of holistic healing, which is central to cancer prevention and healing.[1]

Many people aren't aware of this, but before Hippocrates, medicine was mostly a hodgepodge of tradition, superstition, and magic—not exactly the type of thing you'd want to subject your children to in a life-threatening situation. Many folks erroneously believed that disease was some kind of punishment from the gods, and that the only remedy was basically to pray and hope for the best. Factors like diet, exercise, sanitation, and living habits weren't even on the radar with regard to health, and very few people, if any, specialized in trying to treat illness with actual medicine.

It was the Wild West of health until Hippocrates came along and changed everything. Thanks to his sweeping influence, we now have doctors who serve as educated medical professionals and rely on sound scientific principles formed through clinical testing and rational observation rather than just folklore. There's *order*, in other words, to the way we treat disease today, and Hippocrates is credited as the pioneering mind who first got the ball rolling.

These and other contributions by Hippocrates to modern medicine were enormously positive in the way they created structure and standardization in medical practice. But as you'll soon see, the story does not have a happily-ever-after fairy-tale ending. Outside influences would eventually corrupt Hippocrates's intent and turn medicine into a profit-generating machine focused on disease management rather than healing.

As we embark on this journey together, exploring the history of medicine and how it has changed dramatically since the era of classical antiquity, pay attention to how disease and health would be continually redefined to push this new agenda. It's important for understanding how we got to where we are today, and why it's so vitally important that we change course quickly.

GEOMETRY, NATURE, AND CLINICAL MEDICINE: THE HIPPOCRATIC APPROACH

Before we get into the here and now, let's take a closer look at where it all started. The philosophy behind Hippocratic medicine centers around a geometrical concept known as the Pythagorean theorem: the square of the hypotenuse of a right-angled triangle is equal to the sum of the squares of the two sides that make up its right angle. In nature, this concept is applied as four elements that make up the physical world as we perceive it—water, earth, wind, and fire.

In the realm of medicine, Hippocrates came up with a concept analogous to the nature application of the Pythagorean theorem that he used as a baseline for his approach to healing. The human body, he hypothesized, is made up of four unique fluids or "humors" that need to be in proper balance with one another in order for health to exist—blood, phlegm, yellow bile, and black bile. Hippocrates also believed there were four elemental conditions to human health: cold, hot, dry, and moist.

As Hippocrates maintained, the whole of human health hinges upon a harmonious balance of these separate but intrinsically con-nected parts, none of which can function properly without the others. Today we would call this approach "holistic" medicine, a philosophy of treating the whole sick person rather than just his isolated symptoms. Hippocrates's methods of accomplishing this might have seemed crazy at the time, but they're many of the same methods that are still in use today in the medical field.

Terms such as *symptoms* and even *diagnosis* have their origins in Hippocratic medicine, which is really just *clinical* medicine in its ear-liest, crudest form. Hippocrates saw medicine as an art, with nature as the artist. In his view, the physician's job is simply to facilitate nature in repairing and healing the body, with the patient and the physician working in tandem to provide nature with the tools it needs to bring about this healing.

Hippocrates himself put it simply and beautifully when he stated, "The art consists of three things—the disease, the patient, and the physician. The physician is the servant of the art, and the patient must combat the disease along with the physician."[2]

The incredible legacy of Hippocrates is also bookended by his timeless code of ethics, which is still highly regarded in medicine today as the Oath of Hippocrates or the Hippocratic Oath. It declares that a doctor's job is to treat the sick to the best of his ability, to uphold the privacy of his patients, to pass on medical knowledge to the next generation, and most importantly, to *do no harm* to anyone he treats.[3]

The profundity of Hippocrates's early medical discoveries would live on long after his death and gain acceptance by many others who came after him, including Asclepiades of Bithynia (circa 124–40 B.C.). This lesser-known Greek physician is credited for pioneering what we refer to today as molecular medicine, and he did so within the larger clinical framework Hippocrates established.[4]

COMPASSION, KINDNESS, AND MOLECULES: THE ASCLEPIADEAN APPROACH

While Asclepiades rejected many Hippocratic doctrines such as the four elements, the four humors, and the idea that nature is benevolent in the healing process, the philosophical underpinnings of his approach to medicine have Hippocrates written all over them. Asclepiades also took the "do no harm" portion of the Hippocratic Oath to the next level with his friendly and naturalistic approach to medicine.

According to the historical record, Asclepiades was one of the first doctors to promote the use of medicinal herbs, light therapy, massage, and exercise within a clinical framework; I'll explain more about these approaches later on in this book. He was also the first to differentiate between acute and chronic illness, which he treated from a position of "sympathy, caring, and friendliness," as referenced in a book about his life entitled *Precepts*, which is included as part of the Hippocratic Corpus.

The Epicurean school of thought was a powerful influence in Asclepiades's life, which explains his emphasis on making patients feel loved and happy during the healing process. It also explains why he rejected the benevolent-nature hypothesis of Hippocrates in favor of a more hands-on approach to medicine; using Hippocrates's art analogy, Asclepiades would have viewed the doctor rather than nature as the artist.

Though his name largely faded into obscurity after his passing, Asclepiades's legacy persisted in the various works of his students, including the book *De Re Medica*. Penned by Titus Aufidius of Sicily, this prominent medical text was highly regarded from the time it was first published up until the 19th century, despite enduring waves of rejection from the various philosophical and religious persuasions of the day.

Many of Asclepiades's theories, including his atomic theory of disease, are still relevant to modern medicine's understanding of disease. And while he likely never would have admitted it, Asclepiades's approach to medicine was strikingly similar to that of Hippocrates in that both men recognized the inherently *holistic* nature of human health and healing.

Dr. Christos Yapijakis, a geneticist, biologist, and researcher from the University of Athens Medical School, summed it up nicely in a 2009 paper he published in the *International Journal of Experimental and Clinical Pathophysiology and Drug Research*:

> The great Hippocrates of Kos laid the basic foundations of medical practice and ethics. The brilliant Asclepiades of Bithynia offered a more realistic and humane refinement of the medical art in ways that only recently have been appreciated. It is time that Asclepiades be recognized for his contributions as the father of molecular medicine and take his rightful place as a pioneer physician next to Hippocrates, the justly recognized father of clinical medicine.[5]

IMMUNOLOGY AND THE FEAR OF MICROBES

Even after his passing around 370 B.C., Hippocrates lived on through his legacy, his ethical and moral values becoming a core component of medical practice throughout the world. The American Medical Association's (AMA) Code of Medical Ethics is fundamentally structured around the ideas Hippocrates first brought to life, including his commitment to "do no harm" to patients and to keep their medical conditions private and secure.[6]

The core tenets of Hippocrates's philosophy of disease, however, would eventually fade and be replaced by new theories, including the idea that germs and microbes cause disease. Known as "germ theory," this philosophy of disease is characterized by the idea that illnesses are "caught" when certain pathogens enter the body and start replicating: if you catch a "cold bug," for instance, your body may begin to develop cold systems as you grow progressively congested and ill.

It's an ideology held by many people today, and it arrived on the scene long after Hippocrates's passing, gaining significant momentum throughout Europe and North America between 1850 and 1920. Differing drastically from the humoral philosophy of disease popularized by Hippocrates and many of his protégés, germ theory would eventually become the gold standard of medical practice into the 20th century and beyond.

Part of the reason why germ theory became so popular is that it effectively eliminated all the complex minutiae associated with humoral and other earlier theories of disease, which require a certain level of "outside the box" critical thinking. No longer would physicians have to consider a host of complex factors that might be contributing to a particular disease, nor would they have to give even cursory thought to the supernaturalistic elements inherent to the Hippocratic theory; when you're dealing with germs, a person either "catches" them or they don't, and it's as simple as that!

"Germ theory encouraged the reduction of diseases to simple inter-actions between microorganism and host, without the need for the elab-orate attention to environmental influences, diet, climate, ventilation, and so on that were essential to earlier understandings of health and disease," explains a historical treatise published in Harvard University's *Contagion: Historical Views of Diseases and Epidemics.*

Truth be told, a whole slew of different germ theories popped up as early as the 1600s, several hundred years before the iteration that most people are familiar with today earned the official title. These ear-lier "animacular" germ theories were poked and prodded by the best minds of the time until a unified germ theory that fit changing societal norms was achieved.

"Germ theory was developed in a social, cultural, and economic milieu increasingly centered on the values of mass production, mass consumption, standardization, and efficiency, all of which were com-patible with germ theory science and popularization," explains the Harvard treatise, fleshing out this key point.[7]

With the root cause behind all disease having been simplified down to just disease-causing pathogens entering the body, the basic tenets underpinning germ theory would help propel to the forefront a whole new paradigm of medicine that would quickly become the standard by which doctors treated their patients: symptom management through the use of patented, petrochemical-based drugs.

"Big Pharma," as we often call the pharmaceutical industry, got its start as a result of germ theory, as did vaccinology, the theory that people can be immunized against diseases through exposure to disease-causing pathogens in the form of vaccine injections. Both concepts hinge upon germ theory's antagonism toward infectious "bugs"; hence their focus on eradicating these bugs with drugs and chemical injections.

Edward Jenner (1749–1823), a British physician and scientist, is credited with having developed the world's first vaccine—a vaccine for smallpox. During Jenner's time, smallpox was running rampant throughout the population, except, as legend has it, among milkmaids who were routinely exposed to cowpox from the animals they milked. Jenner theorized that these milkmaids had somehow developed a unique type of immunity as a result of coming into contact with these cows' infected pus, which he applied in the scientific development of the first government-sanctioned inoculation for humans.

Jenner's fascination with the immunological potential of deliberately exposing the human body to disease in order to provoke an immune response, and thus generate natural immunity, would drive a series of experiments he conducted that were ultimately used to validate his theory. He quickly learned that immunity to smallpox could be achieved quite simply through exposure to very small amounts of it, a premise that would gain credence in the budding world of commercialized vaccinology.

"Jenner published many case studies to ensure the whole world knew what he had discovered," documents the historical society at Dr. Jenner's House in Berkeley in Gloucestershire, England. "The research finally led to the naming of this groundbreaking process as 'vaccination.' The name of the process was fittingly taken from Jenner's research as the word vacca means 'cow' in Latin."[8]

Jenner's ideas weren't all that far-fetched from an immunological perspective, especially considering the fact that some of the earliest historical accounts of immunity date back as far as 430 B.C. There were also several others before him who duly surmised that disease could be avoided through inoculation, though their methods were much more crude and far less effective.

According to the historical record, a man named Benjamin Jesty (1736–1816), a British farmer, tested out his own makeshift smallpox vaccine on his wife some 20 years prior to Jenner developing his own more popular version.[9] Some have even speculated that Jesty, rather than

Jenner, deserves most of the credit for being the first to develop an effective vaccine for smallpox because he successfully treated both his wife and two sons several decades before Jenner even arrived on the scene.[10]

But Jenner was ultimately awarded the honor of being the "father" of vaccinology and immunology, and many attribute this to the fact that he was the first to study the safety and efficacy of a vaccine for smallpox using what we now recognize as the scientific method, an improvement from his predecessors that earned him respected status in a number of educational societies throughout Europe.

Ancient China also deserves an honorable mention on the immunology front, as 10th-century records indicate that physicians at that time were treating patients using an induced immunity method known as "variolation" long before Jenner was even a twinkle in his father's eye. Much like modern-day vaccines, variolation involved exposing people to disease lesions either intramuscularly or through the nasal cavity, which imparted immunity—or as they referred to it in ancient Greece, "exemption" from disease. [11]

There's a reason why variolation never really took off during this earlier era, though: it was never properly standardized, and in many cases it didn't work. The Ottoman Empire tried to adopt the technique as a way to inoculate citizens against infectious diseases like smallpox, but many of them ended up suffering severe side effects or dying due to the crudity of the way the treatment was prepared and administered.

It was Jenner's many improvements to these earlier methods, which included extensive scientific testing, that allowed him to develop what many people now credit him as inventing: the world's first scientifically backed method of safely inoculating people against disease. And for this groundbreaking feat, Jenner's name is now crystalized in the annals of history as the leading pioneer in immunology.

MEDICINE GETS EVEN MORE ANTIGERM

As Jenner was nearing the final days of his life, another prominent figure arrived on the scene who would eventually come up with an even more aggressive approach to dealing with germs. Louis Pasteur (1822–1895), a French chemist, scientist, and inventor you've probably heard of, was such a diehard germ theory apologist that he developed his own unique process to literally "kill" food and beverages, a technique that he and his acolytes believed would make food safer for people to consume.

This killing process is known today as pasteurization, and it involves heating something to a very high temperature in order to kill any living thing that might be lurking inside it, including all bacteria and enzymes. Pasteur came up with the idea in response to complaints by brewers who were dismayed that their beers were prematurely souring, the consequences of bacteria feeding on the living constituents left behind after the fermentation process.

Sour beers, ironically enough, are coming back into vogue alongside the IPA trend in today's world. But back then, the souring process was a big concern for manufacturers trying to produce a consistent, shelf-stable product. Consumers expect this and it isn't possible when bacteria are in the picture, which is why Pasteur began aggressively promoting his technique; when bacteria are dead, food remains stable. And this, of course, gave way to an entirely new approach to mass food production known as food "processing."

Pasteur's biggest claim to fame, though, didn't involve food: it was his saving of the French silk industry in 1865, which was being ravaged by an unknown but absolutely devastating microbial infestation. Ironically enough, the method he eventually developed for dealing with this crisis didn't even involve destroying *all* silkworms, yet Pasteur's legacy would hinge upon the notion of total microbial annihilation in order to protect public health.[12]

Pasteur would go on to develop a number of vaccines as well, including his first for chicken cholera in 1879, and several others for anthrax, tuberculosis, smallpox, and rabies in subsequent years. He would gain international recognition for his successful treatment of nine-year-old Joseph Meister, who was bitten by a rabid dog in 1885, and just three years later he would preside over his own institute, the Pasteur Institute in Paris, which was inaugurated on November 14, 1888.[13]

Each of these accomplishments would help fuel a global renaissance in germ theory whereby medicine became completely obsessed with the idea of germs. Pasteur's landmark discovery that microscopic bacteria are teeming in and on almost *everything* exposed to the open air—and that these bacteria could be destroyed with high heat—would forever change the way people looked at germs and public health.

The most significant change brought about as a result of Pasteur's work is one you're probably quite familiar with: milk pasteurization. Though it took some time to catch on, the heating of milk to kill bacteria gained momentum in many parts of the world. It eventually became a food processing standard post-Pasteur, especially as food safety issues began to emerge as a result of industrialization.

Believe it or not, pasteurization was never intended for use on milk as we see it applied today, though milk processors began to use it en masse once they realized its potential to extend the shelf life of commercially produced milk and prevent early fermentation. Pasteurization also helped cover for dirty "swill" milk, killing off dangerous pathogens like typhoid fever and diphtheria that often crept in due to poor sanitation standards.

Despite its prolific use today, widespread adoption of milk pasteurization didn't come without a fight, at least in the United States. Skepticism about what it was doing to milk, and what it might be covering up in the process, kept pasteurization on the fringes until the late 1800s when the first commercially operated milk pasteurizer opened up shop.[14] Prior to this, some milk producers pasteurized their milk in secret to make it last longer on shelves and to prevent the spread of infectious disease.

It was throughout this critical period of time during the late 19th century and early 20th century that the world saw a major departure from historically recognized views about disease. For the first time, society began to view germs, and bacteria in general, as *harmful*, even though fermentation and culturing of foods using *beneficial* bacteria had been taking place for centuries without a second thought.

IT'S NOT THE BACTERIA—IT'S THE TERRAIN

Bacteria, as you may already know, exist all around us *and even in us*, and science has progressed since the 19th century to the point that we now recognize the existence of both "good" and "bad" varieties, something that Pasteur and his acolytes didn't fully understand. These men viewed germs solely from the perspective of being harmful, which is why they spent countless hours in their laboratories developing methods to eradicate them.

Pasteur's claims to fame, pasteurization and vaccines, hinge upon a worldview that looks at bacteria as a menace. And this worldview is still prevalent today; I'm sure you have friends, family members, and neighbors who are deathly afraid of "catching" a disease if they're exposed to disease-causing bacteria or viruses. But is this fear justified?

Contrary to what you were probably told in school, not all bacteria and viruses are bad. Other scientists who lived during the time of Pasteur strongly disagreed with his theories of disease, and they too claimed to have science on their side. Rather than bacteria being the cause of human ailments, they alleged, it's the *terrain* on which bacteria gains a foothold that determines whether or not a person gets sick.

Despite being regarded as one of the world's greatest scientists and the father of serology (the study of bodily fluids), Louis Pasteur *isn't* the man we should be focused on when it comes to legitimate advancements in our understanding of the way the human body works. The real hero, according to R. B. Pearson in his book *Pasteur, Plagiarist, Imposter! The Germ Theory Exploded!*, is a French professor by the name of Pierre Jacques Antoine Béchamp.[15]

Béchamp, who during his tenure served as a professor of medical chemistry and pharmacy at the University of Montpellier, had a much purer understanding of how bacteria works in the fermentation process, a school of thought that Pasteur wholly rejected in favor of the idea that fermentation is *bad* and occurs spontaneously without cause. This is important because Béchamp and Pasteur would end up taking much different paths in their approach to dealing with germs based on their respective beliefs about the nature of germs.

Rarely, if ever, is he credited for his work in this important field. But Béchamp was a scientific rival of sorts to Pasteur, and the conclusion he came to about germs, based on extensive scientific testing, was much more accurate than Pasteur's. What allows germs to proliferate isn't the germs themselves, he realized, but rather the *environments* in which these germs exist. Béchamp also recognized that germs and bacteria have to originate from somewhere, and don't just spontaneously appear as Pasteur erroneously believed.

Far ahead of his time, Béchamp's understanding of germs turned out to be far more accurate than Pasteur's. Béchamp learned that germs are pleomorphic, meaning they can change size and shape depending on their environmental conditions, whereas Pasteur believed germs remained constant—again, the former focuses on the terrain, while the latter focuses on the germs.

Pearson presents mounds of compelling evidence to show that Béchamp, *not* Pasteur, was the true scientific leader of his time who had the most accurate understanding of the nature of bacteria. And yet Pasteur, who Pearson also claims *pirated and perverted* the work of Béchamp, receives all the credit in most modern history books.

Before I get into the reasons why I believe Pasteur took the limelight, I want to introduce to you another man whose contributions furthered the work of Béchamp by giving the world an even greater understanding of the nature of germs. His name is Claude Bernard, and despite being another one of Pasteur's contemporaries, his scientific offerings couldn't have been more divergent.

Béchamp and Bernard were like the Holmes and Watson of 19th-century germ research. Béchamp uncovered much more about the true nature of germs than had previously been understood, while Bernard filled in the blanks as to *why* germs act and function as they do in various environments. The rewards of Bernard's work include our modern-day understanding of pH balance, for instance, and the effects of an acidic or alkaline environment on microorganisms.

Recognized as the father of experimental medicine, Bernard is the man who coined the phrase "The terrain is everything; the germ is nothing." [16]

This credo flies in the face of everything Pasteur had surmised about germs, and yet its accuracy in navigating the more progressive vein of modern medicine has stood the test of time, and it's the direction I'll be taking you throughout the course of this book. Bernard recognized that germs are only harmful when they're in an environment that allows them to cause harm. If the environment can be kept as such to prevent germs from wreaking havoc, he realized, people wouldn't need to worry about being exposed to them.

Béchamp and Bernard were two peas in a pod when it came to reinventing germ theory for the better, yet neither has received the historical credit he deserves. Pasteur gets all the credit for introducing pasteurization, even though this process was an adjunct to a flawed understanding of the nature of germs. On his deathbed, Pasteur actually conceded that he was wrong, and that terrain is everything—but the damage had already been done.[17]

Pasteur wasn't the only one who, coming from an entirely different school of thought, later changed his mind based on evolving science. Rudolph Virchow, another father of experimental medicine, had spent many years in 19th-century Germany (then Prussia) forging the emerging field of cellular pathology.[18] He too had initially bought into the "germs are bad" mind-set along with many others during his time, yet later had an awakening, confessing during the latter years of his career:

> If I could live my life over again, I would devote it to proving that germs seek their natural habitat—diseased tissue—rather than being the cause of the diseased tissue; e.g., mosquitoes seek the stagnant water, but do not cause the pool to become stagnant.[19]

So the general consensus among Virchow, Bernard, and Béchamp was that germs are a virtual non-threat when the environment, or "terrain," they encounter within an organism is properly suited to handle them. And we're not even talking about the immune system here, which is just one component of what constitutes a healthy terrain; we're talking about the body's internal ecosystem, the overall integrity of which is determined by things like chemical toxicity and nutritional status.

Your immune system, believe it or not, technically operates as a type of backup when your internal ecological terrain fails to fend off germs as a first line of defense. Cell tissue then becomes diseased, attracting more germs, and the immune system responds by kicking into high gear, sometimes with success and sometimes with failure.

Maintaining a healthy internal terrain is your first priority, and boosting your immune system is second. Fussing over germs shouldn't be a priority at all, it turns out, and yet this is where we are as a society today. Pasteur's failed hypothesis about germs being the cause of disease remains the template upon which modern medicine treats disease.

The significance of this from the perspective of cancer treatment and prevention is huge, as you'll soon see, because patients today aren't being told about the importance of maintaining a healthy terrain for optimal immune function. For the most part, they're being told that developing cancer is just a gamble, and that people who get it have no choice but to undergo intensive therapy treatments that, much in the same way that Pasteur dealt with germs, attempt to destroy cancer cells with toxic substances rather than repair the damaged terrain that they've penetrated.

Another failure inherent to Pasteur's theory of germs is that it fails to differentiate between harmful and helpful bacteria. Modern science, despite its many shortcomings, is finally coming around to a proper understanding that beneficial bacteria, often referred to as probiotics, are a critical component of strong immunity. One might even say that probiotics are a critical component of the terrain landscape.

Dr. Michael Lam, M.D., M.P.H., an American Board of Anti-Aging/Regenerative Medicine–certified physician, is well versed in the area of biological terrain, and he contends that probiotic bacteria are essential for maintaining what he describes as "the balance of microscopic interplay between billions of beneficial ('good') and pathogenic ('bad') bacteria."[20] The intestinal tract is perhaps the most critical link in the chain mail of your body's ecological terrain, and it's often the entry point through which cancer gains a foothold in the body.

Dr. Lam also emphasizes the importance of maintaining functional alkalinity, as cancer cells thrive on acidic biological terrain. His approach to health falls right in line with the terrain theory of germs embraced by Virchow, Bernard, and Béchamp, and it's the same approach taken with many of the "alternative" and integrative cancer therapies I'll introduce you to later on in this book.

Western medicine, for the most part, still clings to an improper understanding of germs that rejects the ecological terrain component to health, to the detriment of public health. Millions of people are needlessly suffering and dying on account of failed treatments that target germs, not the least of which include pharmaceutical cancer drugs.

CHAPTER 2

THE FLEXNER REPORT: BIG OIL'S TAKEOVER OF MEDICINE

Medicine has gone from representing a delicate balance of science and art—decentralized, open to change as progress dictates, and expressed in many unique forms—to a one-track system of dogmatic and irrefutable corporate edict. How did we get here? More importantly, *how and why* did medicine change so dramatically from utilizing plants and herbs to help the body heal itself naturally to merely targeting disease symptoms using synthetic, petroleum-based chemical compounds; i.e., pharmaceutical drugs?

To find the answers to these important questions, we have to go back to a paper published in 1910 called the Flexner Report, which dramatically—and for all intents and purposes, *permanently*—changed the course of Western medicine. Powerful corporations and the AMA hired a man named Abraham Flexner to conduct an assessment of 155 medical schools throughout North America. Flexner evaluated the various teaching methods used at each school in order to compile and establish the standardized system of medicine that his bosses wanted to come to fruition.

Before the Flexner Report's publication, what many people now refer to as "alternative" medicine was just plain old *medicine*. Practicing doctors took advantage of an assortment of therapeutic options such as homeopathy, which was taught at medical schools throughout the country. Herbal medicine was also highly esteemed within the halls of higher education, fulfilling its own unique role in the vast philosophical consortium of medical education.

Nineteenth-century medical education was primarily taught in one of three ways:[1]

- Apprenticeship programs where local practitioners would provide students with hands-on, one-on-one instruction
- Proprietary schools where physicians would lecture groups of students at their own privately owned medical colleges
- University training programs where students received a combination of didactic and clinical training at university-affiliated lecture halls and hospitals

As you can see, pre-1910 medical education in the United States varied immensely depending upon the school, and *type* of school, at which it was taught. As was the case with most institutions of higher learning at the time, the pursuit of truth through scientific inquiry took many unique forms, and people recognized this as being entirely normal. There were multitudinous schools of thought and all sorts of approaches to medicine, each with its own veritable benefits.

It was a free-market model of medical education that centered around openness and the acceptance of new ideas—*not* top-down control by a centralized few. The ideological precedent for medicine was one that inherently disallowed the type of easily corruptible disease management techniques that we see so often today, and it's why medicine as a healing art flourished so beautifully during that time.

Those ideas that most successfully withstood rigorous scrutiny were propelled to the forefront of what was generally accepted as sound medical science. The greatest advancements in medicine could be attained by virtually anyone with an inquiring mind and the means and wherewithal to achieve success, all without undue bureaucratic impediment.

During an interview I conducted with him for my film series *The Quest for the Cures,* my good friend Dr. Robert Scott Bell, D.A. Hom., told me something about the nature of medicine prior to the Flexner Report that completely blew my mind:

> At the time of the late 1800s and early 1900s . . . medical schools taught a lot of different things. There were homeopathic medical schools, there were naturopathic schools, there were eclectic, herbal-type medicine schools . . . there was not one way. And what happened was that the Rockefeller and Carnegie Foundations were interested in establishing the one way.

This "one way" agenda soon destroyed the decentralized model of medical education. The totality of medicine was consolidated under the umbrella of a single, centrally governed medical oligarchy, any departure from which would be viewed with tacit disdain not only by those who constituted it but also by those who observed it from the outside. Gone were the days of genuine scientific inquiry, sacrificed to the incoming model of authoritarian medicine, and the catalyst was the Flexner Report.

THE ROCKEFELLER OIL EMPIRE'S GREAT MEDICINE HOAX

By now, you're probably wondering what is contained in this infamous Flexner Report that so powerfully undercut the old way of doing things. The answer has more to do with what *wasn't* included—and more specifically, the ways in which these omissions effectively manipulated public opinion to reject the old style of medical education in America, which was dubbed broken and in need of repair.

Recognizing that the American populace was already fully attuned to the idea of free-market medicine, the Rockefellers and Carnegies, who sponsored the report, knew they couldn't just come right out and say that they wanted to consolidate medicine into a unified system under their own control. They had to figure out a way to convince people that medical education was in need of reform, which they did by promoting the idea that medical schools were ripping people off for private gain.[2]

Many medical schools operated as for-profit teaching departments at colleges and universities alike. They accepted virtually anyone who wanted to learn and could pay, and the curriculum varied widely depending on the school at which it was taught, as well as who was teaching it. Something major would have to change to convince people that this open-source model of medical education was somehow detrimental to society. Yet if this could be accomplished, it would then be possible to abolish the old system and usher in a one-size-fits-all system of medicine controlled from the top down, one that could be easily replicated and taught universally at all medical schools.

The three types of schools I mentioned earlier would have to go if the Rockefeller vision of a more "uniformly arduous and expensive" system of medical education, to quote Abraham Flexner, was to be implemented on a wide scale.

Admittedly, some forms of medical education at the time were, indeed, bunk. But in the background was a covert plan to eliminate many legitimate forms of medicine that would compete with this new system, effectively turning medicine into the dispensation of prescription pills as standardized treatment for an assortment of established medical diagnoses. Prior to the Flexner Report, there was no real pharmaceutical industry per se and no single governing authority dictating the course of medicine. But this quickly changed after the oil industry saw potential for profit in its new idea.

"[The Rockefellers] started finding out through organic chemistry that they could alter oil-based molecules into all kinds of things, and they developed these into patented drugs, or drug molecules," Dr. Bell explained to me. "Now these were very profitable, but in order for the public to accept them—because quite honestly, they're poison—they would have to take control of the education system."

A handpicked group of men led by Abraham Flexner (and to a lesser extent his brother Simon) was tasked with developing a new framework for medicine in North America. Spurred on by the Rockefellers and the Carnegies, in concert with the AMA, this cohort of brilliant yet malleable minds single-handedly redirected the course of medical education in North America. The AMA's lobbying efforts during the second half of the 19th century catalyzed the "rigorous brand of systematized, experiential medical education" Rockefeller and the others envisioned when they pioneered the Flexner Report. Flexner and his elite group were merely pawns used to bring about the endgame.

As they converged during these early days of the 20th century, the cohort, dubbed the "Hopkins Circle," developed a whole new edifice for medical education that, in effect, achieved the goals of the AMA, Rockefeller, and Carnegie: a major success for the big boys, and an incalculable loss for Americans, not to mention the various medical schools that were put out of business. Here's what the editors of JAMA (the Journal of the American Medical Association) declared in 1901 about their goals concerning medical education: "It is to be hoped that with higher standards universally applied their number will soon be adequately reduced, and that only the fittest will survive."

These consolidators saw it as a *good* thing that their efforts would result in a major narrowing of the playing field when it came to medical education. In fact, the elimination of competing medical philosophies was the goal all along, and it's what would later allow for major institutions like the Johns Hopkins University School of Medicine—which many today consider the gold standard of science-based medical education—to supplant the entirety of medicine.

"[These interests] would get a hold of the education system and create a medical monopoly via basically eliminating all competition to patent petrochemical medical education," says Dr. Bell. "That's the Flexner Report of 1910, [as] it became known. Abraham and Simon Flexner were hired to do this; it was a pre-ordained commissioned report."

Abraham Flexner, a mascot of sorts, represented this new movement toward centralized medicine. With financial help from his older brother Simon, a pharmacist who at one point also served as head of the Rockefeller Institute, as well as from John D. Rockefeller himself, Flexner spent more than a year and a half traveling the world and penning opinions on what needed to be changed in order to achieve the goals of the cabal. In Europe he gained a treasure trove of insights into the way education was modeled there. He compiled this knowledge into a work he titled *The American College*, which quickly caught the attention of the then head of the Carnegie Foundation, Henry S. Pritchett.

After reading the book, which aligned with his own group's outlook on education reform, Pritchett invited Flexner to assess the landscape of medical education throughout North America and develop a treatise. Flexner's expertise, however, wasn't at all related to medicine—he had previously been a schoolteacher—and this is precisely why Pritchett chose him for the job. "They perceived the problem of medical education as a problem of education and believed a professional educator was better qualified to address this dimension of the problem," explains

Dr. Thomas P. Duffy, M.D., in his 2011 paper *The Flexner Report—100 Years Later.*[3]

Of specific concern to those trying to eliminate the old educational model was the plethora of medical schools operating on the fringes of what would be considered even rudimentary best practices in medicine. The AMA likewise expressed concern about this—at least *publicly* for the purpose of swaying popular opinion. In the eyes of Flexner's various acolytes and protégés, students enrolled in these substandard medical programs were diluting the pool of qualified physicians, thus setting back the profession.

Duffy's article explains Flexner's role as a change agent in this way: "An unflattering but not necessarily inaccurate description for Flexner's assignment was that he was to be the hatchet man in sweeping clean the medical system of substandard medical schools that were flooding the nation with poorly trained physicians."

A major constituent of Flexner's philosophical position on medical education was his newfound affinity for the German model, which he picked up during his travels and studies abroad. It required all budding students of medicine to undergo rigorous scientific training in a laboratory setting prior to even stepping foot in a university hospital system for clinical training. The German model of medicine was already in use at Johns Hopkins, so it was an easy sell, if for no other reason than simple precedent. But Flexner's alignment with science as the "animating force in the physician's life" would become his claim to fame in recalibrating medical education in America, and helping transform it from an art into rote procedure.[4]

What Flexner helped accomplish, in effect, was the unification of science and medicine within a German-inspired educational paradigm that was both embraced and pushed by Carnegie, Rockefeller, the AMA, and the other influential power brokers of the day. Consequently, medicine was transformed, almost overnight.

PROFESSIONALISM: A CONVENIENT CLOAK FOR CORPORATE MEDICINE

As I mentioned earlier, what made Flexner the perfect candidate for the position of change agent to usher in this new model of medicine was that he wasn't a physician himself, yet he understood the ins and outs of education from the perspective of what Rockefeller et al. wanted to see applied specifically to *medical* education. The crafters who envisioned this dramatic transformation recognized that it would create waves within the existing paradigm of medical education, and thus used a nonphysician who had an obsession with the German pedagogic style of medical education as their go-to guy. And it worked out exactly the way it was intended, resulting in:[5]

- A major reduction in the number of medical schools throughout North America
- A major increase in accreditation requirements at teaching facilities; e.g., mandatory teaching hospitals, laboratories, and high-tech equipment
- A whole new litmus test for what qualified as a "legitimate" medical school; e.g., meeting certain expense minimums and having a certain number of facilities
- New laws governing what constitutes a proper science-based medical education
- A complete takeover of medical education by Johns Hopkins–inspired medical schools that were strategically placed throughout the country

The minimum-funding-threshold component of the plan created a convenient back door for the takeover, ensuring that donor and special interest dollars could be used to steer the direction of education at all "certified" medical schools. It was a brilliant scheme, disguised behind the stated goal of making medical education more "professional."

Carnegie Foundation president Henry Pritchett's introduction to the Flexner Report reveals the lengths to which the forces who paved the way for its publication were willing to go in using the push for "professionalism" as an excuse for the overhaul. Pritchett wrote that professionalism, at least as he personally defined it, was a "duty," one that would have to be closely guarded to ensure it remained consistent with the definition he put forth: "No members of the social order are more self-sacrificing than the true physicians and surgeons, and of this fine group none deserve so much of society as those who have taken upon their shoulders the burden of medical education."[6]

"On the other hand," Pritchett continued, "the profession has been diluted by the presence of a great number of men who have come from weak schools with low ideals both of education and of professional honor."

Pritchett was of the persuasion that less was more when it came to medical education: less *competition*, that is. He praised the upheaval of medical education and the subsequent shutdown of competing medical schools that taught osteopathic, chiropractic, homeopathic, physiomedical, botanical, and various other persuasions of medicine. "The very disappearance of many existing schools is part of the reconstructive process," he writes, adding that the objective is a "constructive" one rather than a "critical" one. "Several colleges, finding themselves unable to carry on a medical school upon right lines, have, frankly facing the situation, discontinued their medical departments, the result being a real gain to medical education."

It all sounds so nice—I mean, who wouldn't want to get rid of all those pesky quacks who were abusing medical education for personal gain? This was the narrative being spread around at the time. Flexner's assessment of the medical school landscape helped flesh out the "problem" that those who tasked him with describing it would use to introduce their "solution": the total *dissolution* of all healing protocols that competed with their own.

Dr. Bell summed it up perfectly during our interview: "Not surprisingly, the basis of the report was that it was far too easy to start a medical school, and that most schools were not teaching sound medicine. Let me translate this for you—these natural health colleges were not pushing enough chemical drugs manufactured by who? Carnegie and Rockefeller."

Ironically, the purveyors of the new system claimed that the old system served the private, rather than the public, interest. They lambasted the supposedly commercial nature of the old medical schools, which were accessible to the common man, while praising the philanthropic nature of the newer, more refined schools that, as Pritchett wrote, were designed to "exclude all the unfit" in order to "furnish a perfect body of practitioners."

If you've ever had to deal with pretentious medical doctors who embrace a "my way or the highway" approach to treating patients, you have Pritchett and his fellow reformers to blame. They were instrumental in turning humble patient care into a type of elitist medical oligarchy, in which anything outside what the system deems worthy of scientific approval is treated with disdain. They're also the reason why competing forms of medicine were dismissed as "quackery," even though many of them were standard forms of medicine prior to this time. Many of the treatment methods that I'll outline later on in this book, in fact, are among those that had to go in order to usher in the new system centered around highly profitable pharmaceutical drugs.

This isn't to say that *all* conventionally trained medical doctors today are damaged beyond repair, or that all forms of "conventional" medicine are necessarily all about profit and control. Many doctors practice integrative or functional medicine, combining the best from the "conventional" side of the spectrum with that of the "alternative" side—there are benefits to both, after all. And many physicians, both academic and practicing, have defected from the confines of the system after discovering truths that opened up their minds to a whole different way of thinking about medicine and health. It is my strong conviction that many well-meaning doctors are simply misled, and some of these eventually break free and go on to do great things, including changing the system in whatever capacity they can.

At the same time, pharmaceutical supremacy is certainly a pervasive mind-set that saturates many of our nation's most prestigious medical schools, and it's often the single greatest barrier to true medical progress. And those who embrace this ideology are often exceptionally hostile to "alternative" medicine because it contradicts what they were taught in medical school. It's not that these competing alternative methods don't work—many of them do! But they threaten the profit and power interests of a tightly knit medical oligarchy that has claimed a monopoly over medicine since the days of the Flexner Report.

"The AMA, who were evaluating the various medical colleges, made it their job to target and shut down the larger respected homeopathic colleges," Dr. Darrell Wolfe, Ac. Ph.D., explained to me about the government's role in this agenda. "Carnegie and Rockefeller began to immediately shower hundreds of millions of dollars on these medical schools that were teaching drug-intensive medicine. Predictably, those schools that had the financing churned out the better doctors—or should I say, the more *recognized* doctors. In return for the financing, the schools were required to continue teaching course material that was exclusively drug oriented with *no* emphasis on natural medicine."

Nearly every single medical school that taught something other than Carnegie and Rockefeller curriculum fell by the wayside due to low enrollment, lack of funding, or both. Funding was probably the biggest issue, because the Carnegie and Rockefeller Foundations spent untold millions propping up the schools that supported their agenda at the expense of all the others.

It's important to recognize that homeopathy, chiropractic, and the many other forms of medicine that were largely extinguished as a result of the Flexner Report weren't in the minority when the report was published, as they are today. So-called "alternative" medicine was the *dominant* form of medicine up until the early 20th century when this rapid transformation took place.

"By 1925, over 10,000 herbalists were out of business," Dr. Wolfe told me. "By 1940, over 1,500 chiropractors would be prosecuted for practicing 'quackery.' The twenty-two homeopathic medical schools that flourished in the 1900s dwindles down to just *two* by 1923. . . . By 1950, all the schools teaching homeopathy were closed. In the end, if a physician did not graduate from a Flexner-approved medical school and receive an M.D. degree, he or she could not find a job anywhere. That is why today M.D.s are so heavily biased toward synthetic drug therapy, and know little about nutrition, if anything."

WHEN MONEY TALKS, CORPORATE MEDICINE RESPONDS

For all their talk about being constructive reformers, the entities behind the Flexner Report sure did a number on the medical spectrum as it existed prior to 1910. If you think of pre-1910 medicine as a vibrant color wheel, the Flexner Report was a giant pair of scissors that cut out all the other colors except a single shade of gray. The report sucked the life out of medicine and turned it into a soulless mechanism of profit generation, all in the name of progress. Some of what the report's advocates claim it achieved indeed has merit, such as improvements in educational standards. The German model of rigorous laboratory training, coupled with clinical investigation and hands-on guidance in a hospital setting, is likewise meritorious in that it helps ensure that only the best and most competent physicians are given medical degrees. But the damage this report did to diversity in medicine far outweighs any perceived good it may have done; after all, rigorous educational standards can be applied to all the healing arts, not just pharmaceuticals.

All the problems the Flexner Report was supposed to address—for-profit medicine scams, proprietary curriculum, and lack of scientific rigor—were the very things that the new system embodied, except now without any formidable competition. The artful nature of true scientific inquiry and investigation was tossed aside in favor of a special interest–driven mechanical model.

In his *Yale Journal of Biology and Medicine* article, Dr. Duffy puts it this way: "American medicine profited immeasurably from the scientific advances that this system allowed, but the hyper-rational system of German science created an imbalance in the art and science of medicine."[7]

This imbalance is obvious in the way post–Flexner Report medical schools are now operated: from the top down. And when the Rockefellers and Carnegies offered up massive cash grants to medical schools, they were not only pushing their special interest brand of medical curriculum but separating doctors conducting research from interacting with patients. For the first time, research faculty at medical schools were offered full-time positions and pay to be curriculum creators for the whole of North American medical practice. Proponents of this model argued that the best scientific knowledge could be acquired by individuals who were free to dedicate their entire lives to research and teaching without the "distraction" of treating patients.

But opponents, including a man by the name of William Osler and his colleague Harvey Cushing, foresaw a number of problems with this model: problems that today have manifested precisely as these men predicted. This separation between research doctors and practicing doctors would create "a generation of clinical prigs" who were "removed from the realities and messy details of their patients' lives."[8] The constant pursuit of advanced knowledge by doctors who only conduct research and teach in the university setting would be disastrous for patients treated by practicing physicians taught according to this educational model, whose priority shifted from the humble dealings and nitty-gritty of patient care to trying to rise to the highest ranks of medical knowledge in an institutional setting.

Worse, this shift created two separate and disjointed classes of physician: the highly paid, tenured ones doing the bidding of the medical oligarchy at approved medical schools, and the ones dispensing to their patients what they learn at these schools, which today are almost completely centered around high-profit pharmaceuticals.

Monopolistic medicine quickly became the new "gold" standard, regardless of what anyone had to say about it, and over time the old models of medical practice faded into obscurity, allowing the various rewriters of history the opportunity to shield the machinations of the Rockefellers, the Carnegies, and the AMA from scrutiny by subsequent generations.

One of my goals as I take you on this important journey is to give you fresh insight into the *true and lost* history of medicine, and the ways in which this former art form was hijacked by special interests and turned into a profit-generating machine. As you equip yourself with this knowledge, you'll better understand *why* the alternative methods I'll divulge later on aren't even on the radar screens of many of today's practicing physicians.

RIFE, HOXSEY, FITZGERALD, AND WILK CHALLENGE THE SYSTEM

With the elimination of virtually all competing medical curricula by about the mid-20th century, the new medical system in America was well on its way to achieving total dominance. All that remained was to deal with the competing medical therapies in place before the Flexner Report was published and those that would pop up in its aftermath, much to the chagrin of the establishment. A full-fledged crusade to suppress all *real* cures for disease would have to be launched to protect the pharmaceutical-centric system from any real competition. Recognizing that nobody would agree to take chemical drugs if cheaper, safer, and much more effective natural remedies were available in the mainstream, the medical oligarchy had to get busy knocking these out, one by one.

A conspiracy between Big Oil and Big Pharma arose because these entities are basically *one and the same:* synthetic drugs were manufactured from petroleum derivatives sourced through John D. Rockefeller's Standard Oil monopoly. Rockefeller and his coconspirators would stop at nothing to maintain their grip on both fuel and pharmaceutical medicine, and they were willing to fight against all traditional therapeutics in order to accomplish this.

RIFE'S CURE FOR CANCER AND OTHER DISEASES SQUELCHED BY BIG MEDICINE

One of the most tragic examples of post–Flexner Report medical cronyism is the persecution of Royal Raymond Rife. This distinguished scientist and inventor is credited by those preserving and defending his legacy with discovering that every disease microbe has its own unique electronic signature, and that this signature can be neutralized or "devitalized" in order to cure the disease the microbe causes. Ironically enough, Rife studied at the prestigious Johns Hopkins University in Maryland, a by-product of the Flexner Report's repositioning of American medicine. But Rife's brilliant mind led him to embark on a much different scientific journey that would lead to some truly groundbreaking discoveries in the field of bioelectric medicine.

Rife's many inventions include the world's first heterodyning ultra-violet microscope, also known as the universal prismatic microscope, which contained an astounding 5,682 unique parts and was capable of magnifying objects to 60,000 times their actual size. Rife also came up with the concept of a micro-dissector and a micro-manipulator, discoveries that were instrumental in furnishing many fields of emerging research and technology with the functional tools of their trades.[9]

Rife's universal microscope allowed scientists to see actual, live viruses and bacteria in their true, animated color profiles, and at magnification levels needed for advanced study. This capacity piqued Rife's interest in the potential medical ramifications of being able to closely study both viruses and bacteria, which he theorized, based on his earlier research, could be eradicated with radio-frequency energy.

One of Rife's initial observations upon looking at *Bacillus coli* (*B. coli*) bacteria through his advanced microscope was that it contained its own unique electronic signature, which he discovered could be manipulated to send these particular bacteria into shutdown mode. Other bacteria and viruses, he would later learn, also had electronic signatures, which got him thinking: What if customized frequencies could be developed for each known pathogen in order to destroy that pathogen, and possibly cure the particular disease associated with its infection? After many years of painstaking research, Rife learned that by identifying, isolating, and matching an infectious organism's signature with electro-frequency energy, it was fully possible to destroy it in order to cure disease.

Rife used special tools to send vibrational frequencies into viruses and bacteria to see how they would respond. Using this data, he successfully identified the Mortal Oscillatory Rate (MOR) of each individual microbe, allowing him to fine-tune his special "Beam Ray" to match their respective resonant wavelengths. One historical source explains the process this way: "Just as the resonant frequency which shatters a wine glass can only shatter that type of glass, so Rife's frequencies destroy only disease organisms with the exact same pattern of oscillation."[10]

This discovery was especially relevant with regard to cancer; Rife is credited as the first to discover a virus associated with this leading killer. It took him about 20,000 unsuccessful tries before he identified it—talk about persistence!—but in the end it was worth it. This newly found virus, which he dubbed *Cryptocides primordiales*, became the means through which he would identify a viable cure.

After discovering the precise MOR for *C. primordiales*, Rife was able to demonstrate that his technique worked not only *in vitro* on his laboratory slides, but also *in vivo* on animals—and later in human cancer patients. Rife's finely tuned Beam Ray machine saw similar successes with many other germs as well, prompting his friend Milbank Johnson, M.D., a professor of physiology and clinical medicine at University of Southern California, to push him to the next level of research and development. Dr. Johnson convinced Rife to work alongside a research committee made up of some of the best and brightest minds of the time to conduct experiments on the cancer virus in humans. In 1934, they brought in 16 terminally ill patients, all of whom were successfully cured within three months utilizing the Rife protocol—all without causing *any* harmful side effects.

HOXSEY CLINICS SHUT DOWN BY FDA, AMA, AND NCI

More than 2,000 miles away in rural Illinois, the boisterous great-grandson of a humble veterinarian took a much different approach to curing cancer naturally, though his eventual fate would turn out to be much the same as Rife's. Harry Hoxsey inherited special herbal wisdom from his great-grandfather John, who happened to observe that one of his sick horses, which he had put out to pasture to die, fully recovered after munching on some herbs it found in a field.

According to Hoxsey's personal account in his autobiography, *You Don't Have to Die!*, great-grandfather John gathered samples of the herbs he saw the horse eat, studied and experimented with them intently, and came up with three formulations that would serve as a remedy for humans suffering from cancer: an herbal liquid formula, a powder, and a topical salve. A highly intelligent and outgoing man, young Harry saw incredible promise in the formulas his great-grandfather passed down through the family. Harry had seen his father, also named John, use the herbal blends on human patients in secret. This eventually prompted him to start some 17 clinics where the Hoxsey Tonic, as it was called, could be administered to human patients.

Based on a Native American elixir that contained many of the same ingredients, Hoxsey's internal formula blended red clover blossom, licorice root, buckthorn bark, burdock root, stillingia root, poke root, barberry root, Oregon grape root, cascara sagrada bark, prickly ash bark, and wild indigo root. Later versions of the formula also contained sea kelp, which complemented the potassium iodide that was administered alongside the tonic itself.

Though he wasn't a doctor, and neither was his father, Harry recognized that while his great-grandfather's tonic wasn't necessarily a miracle cure, each of its constituents worked in tandem to help restore balance to body chemistry, the lack of which can lead to systemic toxicity and chronic illnesses. Harry saw cancer in particular as one of the conditions resulting from this imbalance, writing that it "occurs only in the presence of a profound physiological change in the constituents of body fluids and a consequent chemical imbalance in the organisms." In other words, metabolic inconsistencies that lead to diseases like cancer are effectively normalized when treated with the herbs found in the Hoxsey Tonic, a fact later affirmed in a book entitled *Plants Used*

Against Cancer written by Jonathan Hartwell, one of the founders of the National Cancer Institute (NCI).

Hoxsey's external tonic was a red paste containing the red sap extracted from bloodroot (*Sanguinaria canadensis*), a common wildflower, along with zinc chloride and antimony sulfide. It was an adaptation of an earlier healing paste made by Dr. J. W. Fell at Middlesex Hospital in London during the 1850s, which was likewise inspired by even older pastes dating back to pre-colonial America.

"The Hoxsey herbs have long been used by Native American healers to treat cancer, and traveling European doctors picked up the knowledge and took it home with them to treat patients," explains Richard Walters in a 1994 essay that he wrote for *The Herb Quarterly* that was also published in his book *Options: The Alternative Cancer Therapy Book*. "The root stock of blood-root, a spring-blooming flower, contains an alkaloid, sanguinarine, that has powerful anti-tumor properties. . . . According to eminent botanist James Duke, Ph.D., of the United States Department of Agriculture, all of the Hoxsey herbs have known anti-cancer properties."[11]

The Hoxsey protocol is both simple and highly effective, which is why it became popular very quickly. The herbal concoction's ability to strengthen immunity and detoxify waste and toxins from tumors, causing them to necrotize, was appealing to cancer patients who were apprehensive about chemotherapy and radiation, and all the nasty side effects these treatments cause.

Harry Hoxsey's clinics were a rousing success—except for one small problem: his protocol didn't fit the narrative of the American medical establishment. Consequently, he faced frequent persecution at the hands of the state. Historical records indicate that Harry was arrested more than 100 times for allegedly practicing medicine without a license, and his tonics were eventually forced out of the limelight. His popularity among his patients, however, most of whom were cured using the protocol, as well as legislators, judges, and even other doctors, helped protect Harry from ever being convicted of his alleged crimes—at least for a time. Nearly everyone who looked at the evidence, including those who were opposed to the Hoxsey Tonic initially, had a change of heart after witnessing its successes firsthand.

An independent group of 10 doctors who probed Hoxsey's Dallas clinic in 1954 and pored through hundreds of case histories and testimony concluded that Harry and his team of healers was "successfully treating pathologically proven cases of cancer, both internal and external, without the use of surgery, radium or x-ray." They went on to praise the work being done at the Hoxsey Clinics, declaring that the treatments offered there were "superior" to conventional methods, and that everything should be done to bring the treatment to all Americans. But this never happened, thanks in part, according to Harry Hoxsey, to the influence of Dr. Malcolm Harris, a Chicago surgeon and later president of the AMA.

Dr. Harris offered Hoxsey cash to hand over control of the protocol to the AMA, but Hoxsey refused. He was never in it for the money and even offered the Hoxsey Tonic to patients for free if they couldn't afford it. He simply wanted to help people. But the AMA, in concert with various other federal agencies, wouldn't allow this treatment to gain any more attention. So they filed lawsuits against Hoxsey, and even sent the Food and Drug Administration (FDA) against him, a move that would lead to the forced shutdown of all Hoxsey Clinics by the 1960s.

Esquire magazine planned to run a hit piece on Hoxsey and his tonic, sending reporter James Burke to expose the "quackery" in which Harry was supposedly engaged. But as Burke investigated the man and his clinics, looking for any reason to discredit him, he came to a much different conclusion: Harry Hoxsey was not only successfully treating patients, but he was doing so out of the kindness of his heart, treating and housing many of his less privileged patients without charging them a penny. Burke became one of Harry's strongest advocates, writing the article from a very different perspective. He called it "The Quack Who Cured Cancer." *Esquire* never published it.

In the years that followed, the FDA shuttered every Hoxsey Clinic in the U.S., forcing Harry to open up new clinics in Mexico that, fortunately for cancer patients, still operate to this very day. They've been renamed at his request; the headquarters in Tijuana is now called the Bio Medical Center, and it operates just across the border from San Diego beyond the reach of U.S. regulators.

FITZGERALD EXPOSES MEDICAL CRONYISM

Just one year prior to the independent panel's vetting of Harry Hoxsey's work in 1954, a congressional committee was established to investigate the AMA's role in obstructing the use of not only his but many other natural cancer treatments available in the U.S. Congressman Charles Tobey of Massachusetts commissioned a man named Benedict Fitzgerald as special counsel to this committee to investigate the alleged improprieties and compile a report based on his findings.

The resulting Fitzgerald Report's conclusions, which were officially published in the *Congressional Record* on August 3, 1953,[12] shook the very foundations of the medical establishment's encroachments. Its purpose was to assess the state of cancer medicine during this critical time in American history, and more specifically to uncover any foul play in the free flow of medical knowledge and therapeutics: foul play that Fitzgerald both affirmed as true and disclosed with remarkable boldness. In his report to Senator William Langer of North Dakota, Fitzgerald offered a damning indictment of the ruling medical class, which he pegged as engaging in an active conspiracy to suppress natural treatments and cures. He looked at a number of controversial cancer treatments, including the Hoxsey Tonic, and determined that the AMA in its witch hunt had been "hasty, capricious, arbitrary, and outright dishonest" in declaring these treatments ineffective.

Fitzgerald also named names, including that of Dr. J. J. Moore, the treasurer of the AMA at the time who, Fitzgerald wrote, likely involved the AMA and other alphabet soup agencies "in an interstate conspiracy of alarming proportions. . . . Behind and over all this is the weirdest conglomeration of corrupt motives, intrigue, selfishness, jealousy, obstruction, and conspiracy that I have ever seen," Fitzgerald wrote with blistering honesty.

Specifically with regard to Harry Hoxsey and his clinics that had been forcibly shuttered by the FDA as a result of AMA pressure, Fitzgerald reported that Hoxsey was no more guilty of fraud than were the many patients he cured. Hoxsey's primary antagonist, AMA head Dr. Morris Fishbein, was also wrong in declaring Hoxsey a "quack" and a "charlatan," as well as in claiming his treatments were fraudulent when they had certifiably helped hundreds of patients overcome cancer.

Hoxsey won a major court case against Dr. Fishbein, who reluctantly admitted to never having practiced medicine a day in his life and thus couldn't speak authoritatively to the therapies he had attacked. After hearing from a panel of pathologists, radiologists, physicians, surgeons, and scores of witnesses in Hoxsey's defense, the jury agreed that Dr. Fishbein was hopelessly in error.

"The jury . . . concluded that Dr. Fishbein was wrong; that his published statements were false, and that the Hoxsey method of treating cancer did have therapeutic value," Fitzgerald wrote, noting that those who defended Dr. Fishbein's position actually admitted, on the record, that conventional cancer therapies like radiation could *cause* cancer. "This view is supported by medical publications, including the magazine entitled 'Cancer,' published by the American Cancer Society, May issue of 1948," he added.

If this evidence wasn't enough, Fitzgerald listed the names and addresses of patients who, according to independent but scientifically sound pathological assessment, had been cured of their cancers after being treated at Hoxsey's clinics. He also provided a summary of statements from many of the leading medical scientists of the day validating that surgery and radiation-based treatments for cancer weren't effective and caused considerable harm to patients. "While there are some who still believe in the efficacy of radiation as a cure, my skepticism with regard to its value is being increasingly substantiated," reads part of the transcript from hearings held in 1946 before the 79th Congress, which was considering a bill to authorize an expenditure of $100 million for cancer research. In 1939 the great British physiologist Sir Leonard Hill wrote: "Large doses (of gamma and hard X-rays) produce destruction of normal tissues such as marrow and lymphoid tissue, leucocytes and epithelial linings, and death ensues."

Fitzgerald unabashedly affirmed the benefits of Hoxsey's treatments in his report, along with those of several others like him who were the target of AMA persecution, while also providing copious evidence that the establishment's treatments were inferior and dangerous. He warned against the monopolistic forces that were trying to squelch their competition, and argued in favor of a free-market medicine model whereby patients, doctors, researchers, and scientists would be legally protected in pursuit of their respective medical approaches.

The AMA and the American Cancer Society (ACS), both of which had been aggressively peddling the lie that radium, X-ray therapy, and surgery are the only recognized treatments for cancer, were the main target of Fitzgerald's scathing indictment of America's increasingly broken medical system. And their control over medicine, fueled by special interest money from both private and public sources, was the disease in need of a cure.

The "greatest hoax of the age" was the intrepid phrase Fitzgerald used to describe the position of the AMA–ACA attack on competing cancer therapies. And he painted the AMA, ACS, and FDA as nothing short of a medical cabal, holding them to account for hindering, suppressing, and restricting the free flow of competing medical therapies that were cutting into the profits of the "slash, cut, and burn" methods they prescribed. Fitzgerald was also one of the first on the national stage to criticize the medical system's gross obsession with trying to control the dispensation of medicine. Rat poison and arsenic, he noted, were freely available over the counter, but a small tube of mostly harmless penicillin had to be accompanied by a doctor's prescription in order to be legally purchased.

It seems as though Fitzgerald knew even better than those at the AMA the importance of doing no harm, and also doing what's *right*. His conclusions, had they been taken seriously by those with the power to do something about it, would have rooted out the "virus" that was devouring medical freedom and restored access to the treatments of old—treatments that actually worked.

His testimony cut straight to the heart of the matter:

> We should determine whether existing agencies, both public and private, are engaged and have pursued a policy of harassment, ridicule, slander, and libelous attacks on others sincerely engaged in stamping out this curse (cancer) of mankind. Have medical associations, through their officers, agents, servants and employees engaged in this practice?
>
> My investigation to date should convince this Committee that a conspiracy does exist to stop the free flow and use of drugs in interstate commerce which allegedly has solid therapeutic value. Public and private funds have been thrown around like confetti at a country fair to close up and destroy clinics, hospitals, and

scientific research laboratories which do not conform to the viewpoint of medical associations. . . .

How long will the American people take this? It is but another manifestation of power and privilege of a few at the expense of the many.

WILK V. THE AMA: A TESTIMONY TO THE POWER OF UNITY IN OVERCOMING TYRANNY

The chiropractic profession has likewise endured a tumultuous run, facing repeated onslaught from the AMA throughout the last century. As it did to Hoxsey, Rife, and many others, the AMA has set out again and again to destroy chiropractic by publicly undermining the legitimacy of the profession, concealing evidence of its propriety, and manipulating government agencies to view chiropractic in a negative light.

Chiropractic is still around today, but its present existence as a respected profession hasn't come without a tremendous fight. A pivotal factor in its persistence was a landmark lawsuit filed in October 1976 by a doctor of chiropractic named Chester Wilk who, along with three other chiropractors, took the AMA to task for its illegal activity in trying to eliminate the chiropractic profession.

The history of chiropractic dates back to 1895 when Daniel David "D. D." Palmer showed evidence that the nervous system plays a key role in healing. He demonstrated from a scientific perspective that spinal misalignment—or what he called "subluxation"—cuts off nerve communication from various organs (depending on where the subluxation occurs), thus depriving these organs of necessary healing energy. Palmer's vertebral adjustment approach to correcting these subluxations proved successful in an assortment of patients, resulting in a widely accepted, nondrug approach to healing—one that would quickly hit the radar screen of the AMA and other post–Flexner Report entities pushing their own "orthodox" methods as the standard in medicine.

"From its formation in 1895 . . . the chiropractic profession faced a plan of containment and elimination by the American Medical Association (AMA) that continued for nearly a century," explains Steve Agocs, D.C., in an article titled "Chiropractic's Fight for Survival" that was published in the *AMA Journal of Ethics* in 2011. "It took an antitrust lawsuit filed against the AMA in 1976 to reveal the magnitude and scope of the AMA's plan."[13]

Despite rocky beginnings due to minor infighting within the profession—there were several competing forms of chiropractic, after all—chiropractic eventually unified and became its own professional medical organization: something that many other forms of medicine on American soil failed to do, paying the price with their very existence. The profession was forced to vigorously defend its legitimacy throughout the 20th century and even to this very day is challenging the notion first put forth by the AMA that its modalities are somehow unethical and "unscientific."[14] Wilk and his colleagues, after enduring many years of abuse, including unfair licensure laws that put chiropractic at a competitive disadvantage, compiled a solid case against the AMA that repelled its crusade to destroy the profession.

Lawsuits in defense of chiropractic date back as far as the beginning of the 20th century. In fact, a case in 1907, *Wisconsin v. Morikubo*, set an early precedent for the legal practice of chiropractic, differentiating it as a unique branch of medicine distinct from the types practiced by M.D.s and osteopaths, who routinely positioned themselves against chiropractors. That case and a few others laid the foundation for *Wilk v. AMA* in 1976, which proved that the AMA had long been engaged in illegal antitrust tactics against the chiropractic profession, not the least of which included its repeated false accusations that chiropractic was riddled with ethics violations. Another major point in the case that finally gave chiropractic the credibility it deserved was the supposed lack of proper licensing criteria for chiropractors. The AMA had repeatedly harassed chiropractors for practicing without a license, with the result that many of them were arrested and some even jailed. Wilk and the other plaintiffs correctly pointed out that it was impossible for chiropractors to practice without a license since there wasn't even a licensure system in place through which they could attain one.

It was a hard-fought, 11-year battle that would prove critical for the future of chiropractic. In 1987, United States District Judge Susan Getzendanner, after reviewing copious evidence presented by Wilk et al., ruled that the AMA and its codefendants, which included the American College of Surgeons and the American College of Radiology, were indeed guilty of violating the Sherman Antitrust Act, stating that "the AMA decided to contain and eliminate chiropractic as a profession (in order to) destroy a competitor. . . . There are lingering effects of the conspiracy," she added in her scathing judgment. "The AMA has never acknowledged the lawlessness of its past conduct and in fact to this day maintains that it has always been in compliance with the antitrust laws."[15]

But this would eventually change, as the AMA was forced throughout the course of the proceedings to settle three additional lawsuits over its interference with medical doctors who were referring their patients to chiropractors. In 1980, the AMA had no choice but to revise its Principles of Medical Ethics to reflect a new position—which it should have held from the start—that medical doctors are free to choose the patients they serve, the environments in which they serve, and most importantly, the types of practitioners with whom they associate.

The Wilk case is a success story mired in a wasteland of corruption and deceit, but a success story all the same. This critical case became the practical means through which chiropractors everywhere are now able to freely associate with medical doctors, and vice versa, without fear of retribution. When appropriate, the two professions now complement one another in the diagnostic assessment, treatment, and health management of patients.

CHAPTER 3

SMOKE AND MIRRORS

Most of what I've covered thus far deals with what I like to call the "supply" side of the Great Medicine Heist: the people and forces that, from behind the veil, exerted tremendous power and influence in order to force their agenda into medical schools and change the course of medical care. But there's another important factor that needs to be addressed if you're to gain a more complete understanding of how this hijacking was so effective—the "demand" side.

What I mean by this is that seizing control over the medical system and dictating which treatments are "acceptable" and which are "quackery" can be effective only if the people on the receiving end—the ones demanding care—willingly receive it. How do you convince masses of people who are used to the old way of doing things to accept an entirely new paradigm of top-down control when it comes to their health?

The answer is that you mount a disinformation campaign to convince an entire generation of Americans to voluntarily switch out their herbalists for drug-dispensing M.D.s and their nutrition-centric health and wellness ideals for blind reliance on drugs and surgery. One calculating advertisement at a time; one false study at a time; one duplicitous endorsement at a time pushed Big Medicine across the finish line and crystallized its plan for monopoly. It relied on the public's conditioned belief in trusted information sources such as scientists, researchers, and doctors.

As ordinary members of society, you and I were conditioned from the time we were born to believe whatever is told to us by mass media and other "trusted" information sources, whether they be popular magazines, scientific journals, or even just compelling advertisements on TV and in the papers. If the general public could be led to believe that these authorities are in full agreement, for instance, that dietary fat is bad for human health, any evidence to the contrary could be easily dismissed.

The new system of medical education also had the effect of conditioning subsequent generations of students who were immersed in its new curriculum. There was a process of indoctrinating the "educated" into accepting consensus views, with the ultimate result that the "uneducated" general public accepted those views as well.

Remember what I wrote earlier about the authors of the Flexner Report framing the narrative to suggest that medicine was broken and in need of repair, all for the purpose of ushering in their own brand of medical treatments? This same tactic of problem-reaction-solution was also used to soften people up to the idea that drugs and surgery—and in the case of cancer, chemotherapeutic poisons—are the only effective means by which to cure disease.

PROPAGANDA BECOMES "MARKETING": THE EDWARD BERNAYS EFFECT

Before I understood that we, our parents, our grandparents, and in some cases even our great-grandparents were lied to from a very young age about the nature of disease, I too believed what I heard. I remember being afraid of that dreaded cancer diagnosis—which I was taught could strike at any time without warning—and thinking there was nothing I could do to avoid the horrible disease if the fates decided to choose me as their victim.

I now know better, and my mission is to make sure *you* and your loved ones know better too. But earlier in my life, I was ignorant of the truth. I was paralyzed, in many ways, when it came to proactively protecting myself against disease because my health worldview was based on what I saw and heard in the mainstream news, and what I read in my academic textbooks. Maybe you can relate, but the perception I was left with was that disease is largely a factor of *chance*, and if I got sick I needed to see a doctor who would prescribe me a pharmaceutical (or two or three) as the remedy. It was as simple as this in my mind, and I wasn't too concerned with what I ate because I was never really told it was important.

After watching both of my parents and several family members develop cancer and later die after receiving conventional treatments with chemotherapy and radiation, I began to question much of what I believed about our medical system. It was a "breaking the matrix" point in my life that led me to the realization that we've all been sold a bill of goods.

The idea that our modern medical system is actually trying to cure disease and keep people healthy is *nothing but smoke and mirrors*, I quickly realized. Much of the illusion hinges upon the clever marketing tactics unveiled more than a century ago by the so-called Father of Spin, Edward L. Bernays. A nephew of Sigmund Freud, Bernays is credited with a new discovery: people can be easily swayed to support an idea or concept that, absent psychological manipulation, they would otherwise reject after thoughtful consideration.

By preying on people's emotions, you can effectively sell them almost anything. This was the crux of Bernays's newfound marketing approach, which would later be used to sell people on the idea of "modern" medicine. No more would peddlers of products—or in this case, medical paradigms—simply offer up truthful information as a means to inform their potential customers. The new model would involve *deceiving* potential customers by taking advantage of their fears, desires, and lusts. "The conscious and intelligent manipulation of the organized habits and opinions of the masses is an important element in democratic society," Bernays wrote in his formative 1928 book *Propaganda*,[1] which outlines in great detail the way Bernays viewed mass manipulation in the context of forcing new ideas into mainstream consciousness. "Those who manipulate this unseen mechanism of society constitute an invisible government which is the true ruling power of our country. We are governed, our minds are molded, our tastes formed, and our ideas suggested, largely by men we have never heard of. . . . It is they who pull the wires that control the public mind."

Bernays penned these chilling words almost 20 years *after* he made his initial debut in the marketing world with the production of "Damaged Goods," one of the nation's first health-related advertising campaigns warning the public about the dangers of contracting a venereal disease. The project was controversial, and thus had trouble getting off the ground. But Bernays set up a "Sociological Fund Committee" to finance the project and garner support from the public, and eventually it became a reality.

Bernays also helped the Woodrow Wilson administration sell the American public on getting the U.S. involved in World War I, despite widespread public opposition at the time. Using a little rhetorical sleight of hand, Bernays made famous the phrase "making the world safe for democracy," a phrase that hit the American public's ears oh-so-gently-and-sweetly, turning the antiwar tides toward a rousing chorus of support.

What Bernays did, in essence, was to repackage propaganda within an entirely new framework of "public relations," as he called it, making it more palatable to the masses. Manipulation of the public mind was his specialty, after all, and his "engineering of consent" was how public opinion would be swayed to support the emerging system of top-down medicine.

"[Bernays] provided leaders the means to 'control and regiment the masses according to our will without their knowing about it,'" writes Richard Gunderman for Phys.org. "Today we might call what Bernays pioneered a form of branding, but at its core it represents little more than a particularly brazen set of techniques to manipulate people to get them to do your bidding."[2]

Bernays's diverse clientele ranged from major corporations like General Electric and Procter & Gamble to the American Tobacco Company and even a handful of American presidents. His "Lucky in Love" campaign helped make cigarettes appealing to young couples; his "torches of freedom" campaign during a 1929 Easter parade helped convince more women to smoke; and his 1930s smoking campaign led the charge in marketing tobacco as not only a way to lose weight, but also soothe a sore throat!

To help Dixie sell more disposable cups, Bernays founded the Committee for the Study and Promotion of the Sanitary Dispensing of Food and Drink, the sole purpose of which was to convince the masses that the only sanitary drinking cups were disposable ones. No matter the product, Bernays had a technique for selling it, which, as you'll see, was pertinent in the marketing of pharmaceutical drugs and cancer treatments.

Bernays's techniques were so effective at thwarting public opinion that Joseph Goebbels, Adolf Hitler's chief propagandist, borrowed many of them during World War II as a way to rally support for the Nazi party. The postwar climate of emerging consumerism in the U.S. would also apply Bernays's techniques of persuasion, giving corporations fresh ways to market their products.

Perhaps not surprisingly, Bernays gathered a lot of his ideas on how to effectively propagandize the American public from his uncle Sigmund Freud, whose psychoanalytic theories and concepts would be applied in the covert engineering of social groupthink. Psychological manipulation would prove to be the key to unlocking the full potential not of human empowerment, but of human *enslavement*.

Some historians argue that Bernays never intended for his marketing methods to be used for evil, but his résumé of success stories—Bernays is the reason the standard American breakfast switched from toast and juice to bacon and eggs, for instance, to enrich the coffers of a large pork producer—suggests otherwise. Bernays's successors would also capitalize on his methods in order to sway the public to accept, and even *welcome*, the Rockefellers' new system of drug-centric medicine.

The influence Bernays had on the collective American psyche was so damaging that when President Franklin Roosevelt was considering taking him on to help lead the U.S. into World War II, Supreme Court Justice Felix Frankfurter issued a stark warning that resonates even today. Bernays, Judge Frankfurter warned, was actively unleashing a Pandora's box of evil upon the world, adding that Bernays and his colleagues were "professional poisoners of the public mind, exploiters of foolishness, fanaticism, and self-interest."

Gunderman expounds upon this point even further from the perspective of those on the receiving end of Bernays-inspired propaganda:

> By convincing people that they want something they do not need, Bernays sought to turn citizens and neighbors into consumers who use their purchasing power to propel themselves down the road to happiness. . . . Without a moral compass, however, such a transformation promotes a patronizing and ultimately cynical view of human nature and human possibilities, one as likely to destroy lives as to build them up.

This assessment reflects exactly what happened to the field of medicine, in part as a result of Bernays. The groupthink mind-set that Bernays's techniques helped crystallize throughout America made it easier than ever for the emerging drug industry to peddle its wares as the only legitimate remedies for disease.

MASS BRAINWASHING TURNS PHARMACEUTICALS INTO "CONVENTIONAL MEDICINE"

Think for a moment about some of the things you were taught as fact when you were a child that have since been proven false. Depending on your age, you might remember when "four out of five physicians" preferred Camel cigarettes. Or when margarine was a healthier fat option than natural butter. Or when eating fat made you fat.

These are just a few examples of some of the most prolific myths ever to be foisted upon the masses as gospel truth. But there are many others that are still in the throes of debate, including:

- Vaccination is the only way to build robust immunity to infectious disease
- Fevers are bad and should be quelled with acetaminophen (Tylenol)
- Taking an aspirin daily can help prevent a heart attack
- Drinking fluoridated water helps prevent tooth decay
- Chronic pain is a normal part of the aging process
- FDA-approved pharmaceuticals are the only means by which disease can be cured
- Chemotherapy, radiation, and surgery are the only effective methods of treating cancer

Each of these common myths falls into the category of what we would call conventional wisdom: ideas that, regardless of whether or not they're actually true, have gained widespread public acceptance and are thus regarded by the majority of people as "truth" simply due to their popularity.

The idea that conventional wisdom somehow trumps reality is completely illogical, of course; truth is truth regardless of how many people believe it. But groupthink is part of what the social engineers achieved when they capitalized on Bernays's methods of propagandized persuasion, which swapped out critical thinking in exchange for bandwagon acceptance—or as he called it, "engineered consent."

On the flip side, there would also have to be engineered *dissent* against people, and more specifically *ideas*, that defy the groupthink narrative. Both pieces of the puzzle were carefully put into place as part of the pharmaceutical revolution, and soon society was scarfing down drugs at the behest of the new army of indoctrinated physicians, who believed and taught their patients to believe that these drugs would help cure the nation's physical ills.

Doctors who refused to toe the line were soon dubbed "quacks" thanks to the American Medical Association's internal propaganda department, which was established in 1913 to help fulfill the goals of the campaign. Its member doctors and the public were instructed to avoid all forms of "quackery"—all forms of medicine that didn't bear the Rockefeller and Carnegie stamp of approval.

Similarly, the pro-pharmaceutical message was actively dispensed not only in the hijacked medical schools, but also on television, on the radio, in magazines, in medical journals, and even through campaigns launched by government health agencies, many of which were established for the sole purpose of making the new system of medicine appear scientific and authoritative.

It was so comprehensive and all-encompassing a plan that both doctors and patients willingly accepted the new drug treatment approach without question, believing it to be the gold standard of medicine for a progressive society. This appeal to superiority was instrumental in convincing the public that drugs were an advanced form of medicine far superior to all those "primitive" medicines of old, and it was based on the Bernays approach to idea marketing.

Suddenly it was considered low-grade thinking to even consider using herbs and natural remedies in many circles; pharmaceuticals were the medicine of the future. It was essentially "out with the old, and in with the new," and the tactic worked quite effectively across the full spectrum of social strata. The federal government also contributed to this mass deception with Roosevelt's signing of the Food, Drug, and Cosmetic Act in 1938, which created a whole new apparatus for governing which medicines were considered "safe and effective."[3]

Pharmaceuticals were already trickling out of the pipeline prior to this. But Roosevelt's new law sent the burgeoning pharmaceutical industry into overdrive, apportioning to it vast new powers to ensure drug-based therapies remained at the top of the pile. "Big Pharma" was birthed right alongside the freshly provisioned FDA, and each would help maintain the other's existence.

The drug industry continued producing its drugs with the blessing of both the medical schools and the media that advertised its products, and the FDA granted its approval for these drugs, helping to create an illusion of credibility. Remember Bernays's tactic of creating committees to give authoritative clout to his clients' otherwise unpopular ideas? This is what the FDA and Roosevelt's legislation effectively did for pharmaceuticals.

Most people at the time didn't know where pharmaceuticals actually came from, why they replaced traditional therapies of more natural origins, or how pharmaceutical curriculum made it into virtually all medical schools. All they knew was that drugs had arrived, and because of the barrage of propaganda they were forced to endure, they believed that drugs were somehow superior to everything else.

Even the science journals became compromised when they started getting flooded with industry-funded studies sandwiched between advertising for, you guessed it, pharmaceuticals. Suddenly chemical drugs were *everywhere*, and this onslaught of in-your-face drug promotion created a bandwagon effect throughout society.

Dr. Russell Blaylock, a renowned medical doctor and retired neurosurgeon, told me all about how this works specifically with regard to cancer drugs, and I'll delve more into that later. Dr. Blaylock is featured throughout my most recent documentary series, *The Truth About Cancer: A Global Quest*. According to Blaylock:

> These pharmaceutical companies will have written for them "ghost" articles, and what they'll do is they'll get this company that writes articles that look just like beautiful medical articles with all the graphs and charts and numbers and references, and they'll write this article without any authors for the study because they wrote it. They'll then go to an oncologist that's very well known and say, wouldn't you like to put your name on this article? And if you do, it's going to be in a very prestigious journal—in the *New England Journal of Medicine* or some oncology journal that's very prestigious.
>
> A lot of these people attempt this because it puts their name even further out front, so they'll say, yeah, put my name on it. And so they'll put a string of names on the article who had *nothing* to do with writing it, and nothing to do with the study, and they'll end up in a very prestigious journal. Well these journals they choose are the ones that affect how doctors behave and how they treat patients.

They'll read this article, not knowing it's a ghost article, and say, gee, they've gotten tremendous responses, and there are hardly any complications. And so they'll order the drug and tell the patient the same thing they got out of that article. There's hardly any complications, patients are doing very well, and there's a good chance that this could cure you.

This pretty much sums up how pharmaceutical drugs *in general* have made powerful inroads into the medical community: through fraud, deception, and the rest of the tactics I've outlined as representing nothing but smoke and mirrors.

What was always considered "conventional" medicine prior to this pharmaceutical revolution was suddenly cast aside as an "alternative" adjunct to the "real thing"—as if plants, herbs, and nutrients are on the fringe of what the human body *actually* needs for health and wellness. This was the linchpin in the gutting and reinvention of mainstream medicine.

PHARMACEUTICALS AND VACCINES DERIVED FROM CHEMICAL WEAPONS

The truth of the matter is that a diseased human body isn't deficient in chemicals, despite what Big Pharma would have us all believe— it's deficient in *nutrients*. Yet this truth slowly faded into obscurity as the pharmaceutical industry continued its quest to monopolize the entirety of American medicine, pumping tens of millions of dollars into deceptive advertising, phony scientific studies, duplicitous research, and various other forms of propaganda.

The American public was sold a bill of goods, and perhaps the most unfortunate aspect of this is the fact that *few people are even aware that it happened*. The history of the drug industry's rise to power slipped into the twilight, as did the history of *how* the drug industry developed many of the drugs it was now peddling. As it turns out, many pharmaceuticals are offshoots of various chemical weapons developed and used during the two major world wars, and some were even tested on prisoners in Nazi concentration camps.

You likely won't find much of anything about this in the standard history books, but many of the earliest pharmaceuticals ever to be developed were hatched in German research labs, including popular analgesics like phenacetin, phenazones, and acetylsalicylic acid (aspirin). Many of Germany's largest drug companies were consolidated into the I.G. Farben conglomerate in 1925, which, besides monopolizing Germany's drug industry, used slave labor in concentration camps like Auschwitz to develop and test new drugs. A 2009 research paper published in the *Journal of Clinical Pharmacology and Therapeutics* explains:

> With regard to medical and pharmacological research projects, I.G. Farben became involved in experimental programmes using patients from the Nazi regime's euthanasia programmes and healthy subjects recruited without their consent from concentration camps, on whom various pharmacological substances were tested, including sulfamide and arsenical derivatives and other preparations whose composition is not precisely known, generally in relation to the treatment of infectious diseases such as typhus, erysipelas, scarlet fever and paratyphoid diarrhea.
>
> Furthermore, I.G. Farben played a decisive role in the German army's chemical warfare programme, contributing to the development of the first two neurotoxic substances, later known as "nerve agents," tabun and sarin. Some of these activities came to light as a result of one of the famous Nuremberg Trials in 1947, which saw 24 executives and scientists from I.G. Farben brought to justice for, among other offenses, the use of slave labour in the concentration camps and forced experimentation with drugs on prisoners. [4]

After the war, many of these chemical weapons were miraculously transformed into pharmaceutical drugs that were used to treat illness throughout the West, including cancer treatments that involve the use of chemotherapy. Vaccines also made their first appearance around this same time, the natural extension of the new chemical-centric mind-set in Western medicine.

Certain household names in the drug industry such as Bayer, a major manufacturer of aspirin, have their roots in the development of chemical weapons. Germany's Bayer AG produced mustard gas, or sulfur mustard, one of the first chemical weapons ever used in warfare. This noxious chemical is believed to be responsible for killing some 100,000 people during World War I.[5]

In the aftermath of World War I, the Geneva Protocol of 1925 was enacted to prohibit the use of chemical weapons like mustard gas as agents of warfare. But this didn't stop nations from stockpiling them anyway, including the U.S. government, which, during World War II, sent some 70 tons of mustard gas to Europe aboard the S.S. *John Harvey.*

A German air raid sank the ship, but according to the official story, the fumes from the resulting gas explosion led to an "amazing" discovery: mustard gas chemicals may help suppress forms of cancer. Secret research on these chemicals would take place during and after World War II, including in Nazi death camps, and not long after that the first chemotherapy drugs derived from mustard gas appeared on the medical scene.

As I and many others explain in my documentary series *The Truth About Cancer: A Global Quest*, chemotherapeutic chemicals are toxic to *all* cells and human tissue, not just cancer cells. They are a literal poison to the body, poison that is particularly damaging to patients who are already suffering from a disease that leaves them with weakened immune systems.

But the campaign undergirding the push toward chemotherapy—it's the new cure for cancer, its advocates claimed as they indoctrinated the medical community with pro-chemotherapy dogma—prevailed. And before you know it, chemotherapy became the standard treatment modality for cancer along with invasive surgery and radiation, another toxic intervention that damages human DNA and actually causes more cancer.

PHARMACEUTICALS MIMIC AND REPLACE NATURE

Hopefully it's abundantly clear to you at this point that maintaining the illusion of chemical-based medicine's superiority over nature requires a complex web of deception not only in the educational curriculum and the science journals, but also in public relations. It also requires a regulatory system that protects the "intellectual property" of pharmaceutical medicine.

Pharmaceutical companies were granted government protection to isolate chemical molecules from nature and claim them as their own through patents, a process I like to call "bio-piracy," or the theft of the natural world for private gain. Many pharmaceutical compounds have their origins in nature, after all, and in some ways *mimic* nature, though often with a major cost to human health.

"Patented medicines do not belong in human bodies," Dr. Jonathan V. Wright, M.D., medical director and founder of the Tahoma (WA) Clinic, told me during an interview for *The Truth About Cancer: A Global Quest*. "All the giant pharmaceutical companies are holders of patents for molecule after molecule after molecule that's *sort of* like what belongs in the body, just sort of enough to do something, but enough to cause a lot of damage too. If we're going to be as healthy as we can in the bodies we now have, we have to use only the substances and energy that belong in the body, and it makes no sense using patented medications."

It's no accident, in other words, that many pharmaceuticals are intentionally designed to be *similar* to the natural compounds from which they're derived, and yet foreign enough to be "owned" by large multinational corporations. Their isolation from whole plants and organisms, as well as from various chemical and petrochemical compounds, renders most pharmaceuticals a side effect nightmare, and some inherently toxic.

"You can't patent nature, which is why we don't get a lot of money for research in plant medicine," adds Dr. Nalini Chilkov, L.Ac. O.M.D., an author, clinician, and cellular biologist who practices Oriental medicine and acupuncture in Santa Monica, California, whom I interviewed for *The Truth about Cancer: A Global Quest*. "But then they'll make a molecule that looks like the molecule from nature, and then that pharmaceutical company can own it. But that's not really the same animal."

Money and power undergird this pharmaceutical smoke and mirrors campaign, and there's no money and power in nature. Nature is, in essence, entirely *free* because no one person or entity can legitimately claim ownership of it, besides God, and God gives of his bounty freely and without prejudice. Patented medicine, on the other hand, is mankind's attempt to play God by controlling the means to health and human destiny. It does nobody except those at the very top of the pyramid any favors, yet it's the model that rules the day.

As my good friend and former vice president of nutrition at the Cancer Treatment Centers of America, Dr. Patrick Quillin, Ph.D., R.D., C.N.S., told me, pharmaceutical medicine has basically upended the natural order and changed all the rules in order to benefit a few at the expense of the many. "Francis Bacon was the founder of the modern scientific principle," Dr. Quillin informed me. "In 1600, he said, 'nature to be commanded must be obeyed.' And what we're doing in modern medicine is saying, 'We don't care about the rules.' We're going to change the rules.' We know that you need vitamin D and sunshine, but we're going to say, 'We can't patent that, so we're going to try to come up with a drug that bypasses all those pathways.'"

Medical *tyranny* is, perhaps, the most accurate descriptor, and it's a tyranny that I hope to deconstruct with your help.

CHAPTER 4

FORCED VACCINES? FORCED CHEMO? MEDICINE AT GUNPOINT

To even get a pharmaceutical drug on the market, whether for cancer or otherwise, the drug company that manufactured it must file a new drug application with the FDA. Depending on whether or not that company provides clinical trial and other supplemental data with its application, the user fee associated with it can exceed $2 million, according to the latest available data.[1]

Combine this with research, development, and testing costs and we're talking about upwards of $5.5 *billion* in payout to get a new drug on the market.[2] This is quite a hefty sum of cash that only the upper crust could ever afford to pay. And the only medicines considered "legitimate" in modern society are those that undergo this expensive and convoluted process. Based on the structure of the FDA and its governing authority over food and drugs, as provisioned in the Federal Food, Drug, and Cosmetic Act, no food, herb, or other substance can be legally marketed or sold as helping to promote health and prevent disease *unless* it has spent this sum of money, which only the proprietors of patented drugs could ever afford to pay.

It's a system stacked in favor of "blockbuster" drugs that stand to bring in tens of billions of dollars in new profits for their respective manufacturers. Humble herbs and plants, on the other hand, will never achieve similar status because, as I mentioned earlier, there's no real money to be made with nature, at least not the amounts of money it would take to recoup even just the FDA's NDA user fees, let alone costly R&D, testing, and market positioning.

Since there's no financial incentive to push natural remedies through the many layers of bureaucratic tape that it would take to get them FDA approved, they continue to exist outside the realm of "science-based medicine," even though, in many cases, they work *far better* than FDA-approved drugs. Natural remedies are also considerably *safer*, as I'll outline more later on in this book.

The main point I want you to understand is that the system was designed to accommodate proprietary pharmaceutical drugs owned by private interests, not herbs or any other form of natural medicine that existed before it. Even if a natural herb were to somehow gain FDA approval, it would automatically lose its status as an herb and immediately become a "drug."

Only "drugs" are capable of curing disease and restoring health, after all: the mantra repeated over and over again throughout the 20th century, crystallizing a collective mind-set that all nondrug substances that used to constitute sound medicine are now unscientific quackery. This narrative evolved from mere mind-set to full-on *edict*, with practicing doctors not only being pressured to accept and perpetuate the drugs-and-surgery model of medicine, but also being *threatened* with fines, loss of their medical licenses, or worse if they don't.

MEDICINE AT GUNPOINT: THE CONVENTIONAL CONSPIRACY

This was exactly the plan all along: to turn monopolistic medicine into *militaristic* medicine that would be forced on the people, in some extreme cases literally at gunpoint. We've seen a lot of this type of thing in recent years with children being taken away from parents when the parents refuse to subject their children to chemotherapy, for instance, or clinics being raided for prescribing alternative therapies that aren't FDA-approved.

Though it might seem like a fairly recent phenomenon, this has been going on for years—and it's getting progressively worse. Some of the earliest known cases date back to the time of the Flexner Report when doctors were falsely accused of ethical violations simply for practicing their specialties. But now we're seeing incidents where families are being ripped apart and people are going to jail.

It all comes back to money and control: pharmaceuticals are just too profitable to leave to chance, especially when the alternatives are cheaper and much more effective. The public has to be coerced and ultimately *forced* to use patented drugs or the entire house of cards will come tumbling down, and the system knows it. That's why all other cancer treatments besides chemotherapy, radiation, and surgery are *illegal* in the United States. Anticancer foods, herbs, and supplements are still available, but they typically can't be labeled as such thanks to federal law. Remember: any substance that's branded as treating or curing disease *must* be approved for such use by the FDA, and the FDA only approves drugs, *never* natural substances, for such purposes.

"According to the FDA's legal definition, a drug is anything that 'diagnoses, cures, mitigates, treats, or prevents a disease," explains Sayer Ji, founder of GreenMed*info* and an ally of mine in the truth movement. The FDA has assumed for itself Godlike power, requiring that its official approval be obtained before any substance can legally be used in the prevention and treatment of disease. The FDA's legal-regulatory control therefore is totalitarian and Napoleonic in construct; what it does not explicitly permit as a medicine is implicitly forbidden."[3]

If anything, it should be the other way around. The general public, as well as licensed practitioners, should be allowed to freely utilize whatever substances they choose and shouldn't have to first gain permission from some government agency in order to do so. But this is where we are.

The FDA claims, as the agency's creators did, that these rules are only intended to assure the consumer that drugs "are safe and effective for their intended uses."[4] In other words, the FDA absolutely *must* rubber-stamp medicine or it will be dangerous and unfit for use.

It's that same problem-reaction-solution scenario of social manipulation that I described in an earlier chapter, except this one has had catastrophic consequences for public health. Not only is the FDA refusing to acknowledge a plethora of "unapproved" substances that have been used for millennia to treat disease, but the agency is also failing to protect the public against the damaging effects of the drugs it *does* approve.

As my good friend Dr. Joseph Mercola notes on his website, at least 100,000 people in the U.S. die every year as a result of taking FDA-approved pharmaceutical drugs![5] And these deaths aren't typically the result of an overdose, by the way; many of them result from patients using pharmaceuticals as prescribed, only to suffer horrific adverse events in the process.

Doctors are under a gag order to toe the line or else pay the price. Many who've tried to buck the system have been threatened with having their licenses revoked, and some actually *have* lost their licenses. One of the more notable cases of this is Dr. Andrew Wakefield, a world-renowned gastroenterologist who lost his medical license in the U.K. after publishing research linking inflammatory bowel disease to a common trivalent vaccine for measles, mumps, and rubella. The reason Dr. Wakefield's research caused such a stir is because inflammatory bowel disease is commonly associated with autism, and autism is something the establishment has been working tirelessly to disassociate from having any connection to vaccines. Dr. Wakefield never said that vaccines caused autism, but his research seemed to inadvertently point in that direction, prompting him to suggest that parents forego the combination MMR vaccine in favor of individual vaccines for measles, mumps, and rubella. He never even came close to decrying *all* vaccines, yet he was accused of such, slandered in the media, and stripped of his title in the U.K.[6] This is just one example among many of how the system handles potential threats to its own existence.

It happens with pharmaceuticals, but it *especially* happens with vaccines and conventional cancer therapies. This despite the fact that both of the latter interventions come with known risks that, in some cases, are *permanent and irreversible*. The principle of "do no harm" doesn't seem to apply when it comes to the immune system (vaccines) or a cancer diagnosis (chemotherapy), and this is a problem.

MANDATORY VACCINES: WHAT HAPPENED TO FREEDOM OF CHOICE?

I find it peculiar that some of the greatest public health "achievements," as they're often called—things like artificial water fluoridation and vaccinations—are interventions that people don't really have the choice to opt out of. There are ways to do it, of course, but they're laborious and in many cases so convoluted that most people just cave for the sake of ease. When it comes to vaccines, they've almost always been voluntary like any other form of medicine—unless you're in the military or work in the health care field. But in recent years, legislators have been chipping away at vaccine freedom for everyone else as well, with Senate Bill 277 in California a primary example of how bureaucracy gone wild is progressively stripping us of our collective medical freedom.

Until the summer of 2015, every state in the Union recognized the right of individuals to opt out of vaccinations for reasons of personal conscience, religious conviction, and/or medical need. In California, all three exemptions were on the books until Governor Jerry Brown signed into law S.B. 277, which eliminated the philosophical and religious exemption options, leaving only the medical option.[7] California is currently the most populous state in America, which means the implications of this bill's passage on the rest of the country, especially in light of the massive groundswell of opposition that emerged to counter it, are tremendous. The Association of American Physicians and Surgeons, the California Chiropractic Association, ParentalRights. org, and many others were among the opponents of the bill.

As of July 1, 2016, public school students in California will be forced to take a barrage of vaccinations unless they can obtain a doctor's note indicating a medical condition that qualifies for an exemption. It's a clear violation of medical freedom, parental rights, and most importantly *human* rights because, regardless of whether or not one supports the idea of vaccines, there's simply no denying that *all* of them come with the risk of adverse events. Because of this inherent risk, no individual should ever be forced to get vaccinated against his or her will, *ever*. Yet in this modern scientific age, health authorities are progressively reprogramming an entire generation to accept the idea that not only are vaccines *necessary* for immune health, but *everyone* has to be vaccinated in order for them to work—they often call this "herd immunity."

I won't get into all the nitty-gritty details of why herd immunity is a farce because my main focus with this book is on cancer. But suffice it to say that centralized medicine has pulled yet another fast one with vaccines, which are part and parcel of the Great Medicine Hoax that I outlined earlier. And the same manipulation that's being used to push mandatory vaccinations is being used to sell toxic chemotherapy and radiation as the only means to managing and "curing" cancer.

For those who are successful in navigating all the red tape and opting out of vaccinations that would otherwise be mandatory, there's still the risk of being prosecuted by the state for alleged "child neglect" or even having your children taken away from you. Consider the following examples of how parents are being persecuted by the system for refusing vaccinations for their children:

- In 2003, a young couple from Colorado was forced to have their newborn baby vaccinated for hepatitis B after the hospital where the baby was born determined that the child's mother tested positive for the disease. She didn't actually have hepatitis; the test is admittedly wrong about 50 percent of the time. Armed guards were present as the child was forcibly vaccinated against the religious and philosophical objections of her parents.[8]

- In 2011, a cohort of pediatricians from across the country, prompted by the American Academy of Pediatrics, announced that it would no longer treat children who weren't vaccinated in accordance with the schedule issued by the U.S. Centers for Disease Control and Prevention (CDC). The reasoning? These pediatricians are supposedly worried about the "health of the children," and believe that unvaccinated children put other children at risk.[9]

- In 2012, a Pennsylvania mother was harassed by the local sheriff's department after her disgruntled pediatrician decided to call both the police and child protective services on her for refusing to vaccinate her son. The pediatrician had falsely accused the mother of acting in a "suspicious" manner simply for standing up for her right not to subject her son to vaccines containing questionable viral fragments and toxic chemicals.[10]

- Even parents who succumb to the pressure to vaccinate their children aren't necessarily off the hook when it comes to state interference. Conditions like "sudden infant death syndrome," also known as SIDS, and "shaken baby syndrome" are two "mystery" conditions that authorities claim have no known cause. But research suggests that both conditions may be linked to vaccines.

In 2014, researchers from the University of Milan in Italy published a paper in the journal *Current Medicinal Chemistry* that implicates hexavalent vaccination as a possible cause of SIDS. The combination diphtheria, pertussis (whooping cough), polio, and influenza vaccine, the researchers found, was associated with acquired hyperacute encephalitis of the tractus solitarii nucleus, a cluster of nerve cells found in the brain. They wrote that the vaccine's components may have "a direct role in sparking off a lethal outcome in vulnerable babies."[11]

Then there's shaken baby syndrome (SBS), an absolute misnomer for a disease if there ever was one. When the identifying markers of this condition emerge in a child—subdural hemorrhage, retinal hemorrhage, and/or encephalopathy—that child's parents are blamed, almost as a rule, for supposedly shaking the child so hard that he or she suffers brain damage.

The medical establishment insists that any manifestation of SBS must be a sign of child abuse, but sound science suggests otherwise. Take a look at what Dr. Harold E. Buttram, M.D., a practicing physician and diplomat at the American Board of Environmental Medicine, found after looking more closely at a number of case studies:

> Based on observation and a limited suggestive body of medical literature, it appears that we may be witnessing in many SBS cases the adverse effects from interactions of highly potent vaccines given in combination. These potentially include: Hepatitis

B (hemorrhagic vasculopathies, autoimmune reactions, neuropathies), *Hemophilus influenza* (hypersensitization), tetanus (hypersensitization), and pertussis (hypersensitization, brain edema, and the effects of endotoxin in causing vascular inflammation and hyper-coagulability).[12]

Having to watch your child suffer such horrific side effects following vaccination is bad enough. But some parents have also had to fight the courts just to prove that they weren't personally responsible for inflicting this harm on their own children, adding insult to injury. Some have been successful, but many others haven't—and some parents have even been sent to *prison* after being falsely convicted of child abuse.

One such tragic case occurred in Florida in 2002 when Brian Patrick Herlihy was convicted of killing his son after the child died of subdural bleeding and brain atrophy. Expert physicians who testified against Herlihy failed to evaluate his son's prenatal and postnatal medical records, and duly ignored the obvious link between the boy's serious health problems and the vaccines he was given. Herlihy was imprisoned due to "sloppy and incomplete medical investigations."[13]

Call it "vaccinophobia" or whatever you wish, but there's a major conspiracy taking place with regard to vaccine safety and effectiveness, and few in the government or media apparatus are willing to address it. Considering the only calculable immunity actually conferred through vaccines is to vaccine manufacturers (the 1986 National Childhood Vaccine Injury Compensation Program quietly created a shield around Big Vaccine, sheltering it from liability in the event of personal injury[14]), all the risk falls squarely on parents and their children. So while opting out of vaccines can be a rather arduous process depending on your stage in life and the state in which you live, it's there for the taking, despite being under constant attack. The National Vaccine Information Center keeps close tabs on vaccine-related news and legislation, and has also made available a state-by-state breakdown of vaccine exemption options that I highly recommend you familiarize yourself with for the betterment of you and your family.[15]

By the way, even simple *speech* that contradicts the pro-vaccine narrative is now apparently off limits, with the recent pulling of the film *Vaxxed*[16] from the Tribeca Film Festival in New York a case-in-point example of First Amendment censorship. This telling documentary, which presents a science-based look into the vaccine-autism connection, was scrapped during the final hour by festival headman Robert De Niro, who may have caved to pressure from the industry to keep it under wraps.[17] *Vaxxed* was also pulled from the WorldFest–Houston International Film Festival in Texas after Houston mayor Sylvester Turner decided that the city shouldn't fund a film "encouraging people not to have their kids vaccinated."[18] Mind you, *Vaxxed* simply tells the full, uncensored truth about vaccines, including alleged criminal corruption at the CDC as relayed by CDC whistleblower Dr. William Thompson. Such information is pertinent to parents considering whether or not, or at what scheduled rate, to vaccinate their children.

THE SCIENTIFIC CASE AGAINST CHEMOTHERAPY

Because the medical establishment markets vaccines as a type of preventative medicine, having spent many decades propagandizing the public into believing that chemical-laden jabs, and not the body's own immune system, are the only way to protect against infectious diseases, it's not all that surprising that the vaccine industry has resorted to trying to muzzle free speech in order to protect itself from scrutiny. It's the same scenario with chemotherapy, which sits right alongside vaccines on the shaky ground of deceit. Oncologists are deluged with pro-chemotherapy propaganda from the moment they enroll in medical school until the time they graduate. They receive little, if any, nutrition education, and are basically taught that drugs—or in this case, repackaged mustard gas—are the only means by which to "manage" cancer.

They never talk about a cure, at least not in any sort of practical way other than "one day we'll find it," because a cure would decimate the multibillion-dollar cancer racket of which they're a part—and eliminate the need for oncologists! Here are a few tidbits of truth about chemotherapy that you'll never hear from the corporate media or conventional doctors, both of which work tirelessly to keep people in the dark about what it actually is and what it does to the body:

1. *Chemotherapy causes cancer.* That's right: one of the premier treatments for cancer—and one of the only treatments *legally* accessible to cancer patients—is carcinogenic by its very nature. Chemotherapy actually *strengthens* cancer cells by turning them into stem cells, which are "master" cells from which other cells are birthed. What chemotherapeutic substances do, in essence, is *add* to the army of cancer cells that are already destroying a patient's body, obliterating all the surrounding healthy cells in the process.

   A 2009 paper out of China that was published in the journal *Bioscience Hypotheses* explains how chemotherapy is actually *more* harmful than doing nothing because, rather than attack the heart and head of the beast, so to speak, it actually *strengthens* it, making cancer stronger and more lethal.[19]

   Cancer stem cells are regarded as the hurdle of cancer therapy at least partially due to their intrinsic resistance to therapy. To this end, chemotherapy is widely used for enrichment of cancer stem cells. In contrast to the dogma, we hypothesized that besides enrichment, cancer stem cells could also be induced by chemotherapy in those regions without sufficient drug delivery. Due to the imbalance of the angiogenesis and insufficient blood supply in certain regions of the tumor mass, chemotherapy delivery is compromised in these regions.

But here's the real kicker (with my own emphasis added): "The insufficient drug delivery in turn *transforms the bulk of cancer cells to stem cells* rather than kill them . . ."

In other words, chemotherapy is a lot like the promotion rule in chess, where a simple pawn (an ordinary cancer cell) is able to achieve queen status (a cancer stem cell) by moving to the correct promotion square. Chemotherapy acts as the vehicle, or perhaps the road map, whereby a basic cancer cell is able to be "promoted" to cancer stem cell status. And cancer stem cells are like a *factory*, of sorts, that churns out more basic cancer cells and proliferates more cancer.

2. *Most oncologists reject chemotherapy for themselves and their families.* If anyone knows firsthand the effects of chemotherapy on the human body, it's the oncologists who are treating their patients with it. And an overwhelming majority of them, according to a 2014 study published in the open-access journal *PLOS ONE*, say they would *never* receive the treatment themselves if they were diagnosed.[20] Of the more than 1,000 doctors who participated in the study, an astounding 88.3 percent admitted that they would forego the "high-intensity care" for themselves—this is code for highly toxic treatments like sweeping, immune-destroying chemotherapy drugs—that they routinely administer to their patients, presumably

because they understand just how destructive and ineffective these treatments truly are for the human body. "Our current default is 'doing,' but in any serious illness there comes a tipping point where the high-intensity treatment becomes more of a burden than the disease itself," admitted clinical associate professor of medicine at the Stanford University School of Medicine, Dr. V. J. Periyakoil, in an interview with the U.K.-based *Daily Mail* newspaper.[21] As to why doctors prescribe these high-intensity treatments regardless, she added, "We don't train doctors to talk (to patients) or reward them for talking. We train them to do and reward them for doing. The system needs to be changed."

An earlier survey out of McGill University in Canada asked 118 doctors, all of whom were experts on lung cancer, whether or not they trusted—and would *use*—the chemotherapy drugs they were administering to patients. A shocking 75 percent of them said they didn't and wouldn't.[22] A similar, follow-up survey conducted six years later found that, while support for chemotherapy had increased based on the sampling of participants, nearly *half* of doctors would still opt out of chemotherapy for themselves, and presumably their families.[23]

3. *Chemotherapy drugs are big business.* So why, then, do oncologists by and large continue to administer chemotherapy drugs if most of them recognize just how detrimental they are to human health? The answer is money. Cancer drugs are the only class of pharmaceutical that's administered directly from doctor to patient, as opposed to being *prescribed* by a doctor and *fulfilled* by a pharmacist on behalf of a patient.

Believe it or not, oncologists actually receive a financial kickback every time they prescribe chemotherapy drugs to their patients. Much like an affiliate program, this cash-back allowance, of sorts, incentivizes the most unscrupulous of cancer doctors to prescribe as much chemotherapy as possible because it's how they make their living. "The significant amount of our revenue comes from the profit, if you will, that we make from selling the drugs," admitted Dr. Peter Eisenberg, a private physician who specializes in administering conventional cancer treatments, in a 2006 interview with NBC News.[24] "So the pressure is frankly on to make money by selling medications."

4. *Chemotherapy has a very low success rate.* It has been proven time and time again that the same chemotherapy drugs that are highly toxic and create huge profits for oncologists are *outrageously ineffective* all the way around, offering a roughly *2 percent chance of success* to most cancer patients who receive them. The results of a 14-year study published in the *Journal of Clinical Oncology* in 2004 revealed that among 154,971 cancer patients from both Australia and the U.S. representing 22 different types of cancer, a mere 2.3 percent and 2.1 percent, respectively, survived for longer than five years after undergoing chemotherapy.[25]

TAKE YOUR CHEMOTHERAPY, OR ELSE

If chemotherapy were merely one option among many for cancer patients, it would be slightly less offensive as a state-sanctioned form of cancer treatment. But besides radiation and surgery, it's technically the *only* option that can legally be prescribed to cancer patients as treatment—and if you're a minor who's been diagnosed with cancer, you may not even have the choice to decline it.

Young Cassandra Callender of Connecticut learned this the hard way after being diagnosed with stage III–IV Hodgkin lymphoma in 2014. After receiving her diagnosis and being recommended chemotherapy as treatment, Cassandra, with the blessing of her mother, decided to seek a second opinion. And simply for making this request, she encountered the ugly face of what I call "gunpoint medicine." Cassandra and her mother were told by the state that chemotherapy was her "only option" for treatment, and that if she didn't take it she would die a horrible death. Frightened by the prospect that she might be forced to take this treatment against her will, Cassandra decided to run away from home. But after learning that this decision could result in her mother going to jail, she returned, only to face the most horrific experience of her life.

In December 2014, the Callender home was ambushed by Hartford police along with agents working on behalf of the Connecticut Department of Children and Families, and Cassandra was forcibly abducted and taken to Connecticut Children's Hospital for mandatory chemotherapy treatment. She was strapped down to a table and administered the treatment against her own will and the will of her family. "At that point, I didn't feel like a human anymore," she recalled during an exclusive interview I conducted with her after she was eventually released. "I feel like I've been violated . . . my ankles and wrists were bruised when I woke up."[26] Cassandra was 17 at the time when she was diagnosed, which the state argued put her under *their* jurisdiction rather than the jurisdiction of her own parents.

A similarly horrifying example of gunpoint medicine occurred to young Thomas Navarro, who was four at the time when he was diagnosed with a form of brain cancer known as a medulloblastoma. As with Cassandra's case, young Thomas's parents didn't want their precious child to be subjected to a toxic treatment that doesn't work and has a high probability of causing more cancer and eventually death. So they tried to opt for an alternative treatment offered by Dr. Stanislaw Burzynski (I'll cover Dr. Burzynski's antineoplaston treatment in greater detail in later chapters) that's been shown to be particularly efficacious against brain tumors, only to encounter the same resistance that the Callenders encountered.

"The FDA went to great lengths to prevent Thomas from receiving the therapy, and only after extensive legal wrangling, great expense, and being forced to submit to conventional treatment first did the family finally receive approval to use Dr. Burzynski," my good friend Dr. Joseph Mercola wrote in an exposé of this deeply disturbing incident. "Unfortunately, at that point it was too late. The damage from the chemo was too great, and he lost his battle with cancer at the tender age of six. His death certificate states the cause of death as: *Respiratory failure due to chronic toxicity of chemotherapy.*"[27]

This same sobering scenario continues to play out time and time again with many other cancer patients—with no consequences for the perpetrators and no end in sight.

One small glimmer of hope in all this is that not *everyone* who's tried to escape the clutches of the "cut, slash, and burn" approach has failed in their efforts. Jared Bucey, the "Kid Against Chemo," is a living example of why it's important for *every* person to take a stand—and more importantly, why *every single person reading this book* needs to make a commitment to stand with each other and with people like Cassandra, Thomas, and Jared, to defend our collective right to choose the medicines with which were are treated.

Like Cassandra, Jared was diagnosed with stage IV Hodgkin lymphoma, and after an initial bout of chemotherapy decided to stop it. Recognizing that the chemotherapy poisons were destroy-ing his body—"I felt my body shutting down"—Jared opted to go the alternative route, and he's now earned for himself a clean bill of health.[28] On his Facebook page, Jared tells the amazing story of how going organic, juicing, and perhaps most importantly *detoxifying* his body using an infrared sauna, a rebounder, and routine coffee enemas, effectively *cured* him of his cancer—that's right, *cured*. I'll cover many of the treatment methods he used in much greater detail later on in this book, but I wanted to give you a small taste of what's to come because, despite the fact that the cards are stacked against those who would choose the route Jared did, there *is* hope!

Part II

Cancer Diagnosis, Detection, Causes, and Prevention

CHAPTER 5

CANCER BASICS AND STATISTICS

Imagine for a second that you've never driven a car. Sure, you've seen cars on the road all your life and understand to some degree how they work as you watch them at a distance. But you have no idea how a car engine functions: how the brakes operate, that a car requires the right type of motor oil and routine oil changes in order to run, and in the case of a manual transmission, that the clutch needs to be engaged in order to shift into another gear and slowly disengaged as the gas pedal is pressed in order to accelerate. Now imagine that you just purchased your first vehicle, and the salesman has handed over the keys without explaining to you anything about how to operate or maintain your new ride. Assuming you knew nothing about cars, you probably wouldn't have a clue about how to check your tire pressure, replace the oil, swap out the brake pads, or even fill the gas tank—and if the salesman didn't show you anything about how to operate the vehicle, you probably wouldn't even know how to start the ignition!

You'd be completely lost before you even left the dealership parking lot, which is how many people are when it comes to understanding their bodies in relation to cancer. We all know that some people *get* cancer, and some of us are even aware of the fact that more people than ever before seem to be getting it. But how many of us really know what cancer *is* or how a person develops it, let alone how to effectively *treat and cure* it?

These are legitimate questions worth asking since society is awash in cancer awareness campaigns that, ironically, tell us next to *nothing* about the true nature of cancer, and most importantly, how to avoid it. Our bodies were designed by God to effectively thwart cancer on their own, given the proper environment and circumstances. But I would venture to say that most people probably don't have a clue what this entails because nobody's telling them, especially not those profiting from the failed treatment of cancer with chemotherapy and radiation.

Now, I understand that the medical industry isn't technically the salesman or even the car manufacturer in this particular analogy. If you consider your body the "vehicle" that gets your soul from point A to point B in the physical, earthly realm, then God is the true designer of your "car" and the one who made it to function optimally as is—assuming you take care of it and do the appropriate things to make sure it doesn't break down and fall apart.

But that's just it: from the time we're born to the time we die, most of us are deprived of the knowledge we need to keep ourselves healthy and disease free. The medical industry has basically locked away the "owner's manual" and thrown away the key, leaving the average person starved for understanding as he or she meanders down the pathway to chronic disease and possible early death.

My goal is to help as many people as possible break free from the prison of ignorance and grab hold of their natural birthright, which includes having a proper understanding of how the human body works and what's required to keep it in tip-top shape. I don't want to see another person fall victim to the medical system. That's why I've gone to painstaking lengths to make sure the truth gets out there to everyone who will receive it.

CELLULAR HEALTH, IMMUNITY, AND CANCER

The human body really is an amazing life form unlike any other. It's nothing short of *miraculous* how its many complex parts perfectly inter-act to keep blood circulating, organs functioning, and the immune system operating 24 hours a day, seven days a week. The cellular system alone is so uniquely suited for the job of keeping our bodies alive that it would be an injustice to try to capture the full essence of its abilities in just a few short paragraphs.

I will say that our cells, which number in the hundreds of *trillions,*[1] are responsible for a host of diverse bodily functions. If your body was its own country, your cells would be the collective workforce that keeps it prospering: some cells regulate breathing, others regulate the immune system, while still others gather and dispose of waste. And all of this happens at the same time that cells are processing and converting both oxygen and blood sugar into energy.

As I covered in my earlier work *Cancer: Step Outside the Box*, healthy cells are those that exist in an *aerobic* state, meaning they effectively produce energy in the form of adenosine triphosphate, or ATP, which is absolutely essential for the function of the entire cellular system. In the absence of ATP, necessary processes like cellular repair, protein and neurotransmitter synthesis, and enzyme and hormone production would cease to occur, as would cellular reproduction and DNA repair.

In order for your cells to produce the high amount of ATP required for self-perpetuation and regeneration, certain inputs must be main-tained, not the least of which include healthy diet and toxin elimina-tion. When these are lacking, or when your body gets thrown out of whack due to too much "bad" and not enough "good," the effect is a compromised immune system, which can lead to pathogenic invasion and, in some cases, the growth and spread of cancer cells.

A cancer cell is really just a healthy cell that turned unhealthy as a result of pathogenic exposure, toxins, or some other malignant factor that caused it to go awry. Cells in general are programmed to replicate, and cancer cells are no different: when they aren't taken out by the immune system, they divide and multiply, eventually forming a cancerous tumor.

Believe it or not, our bodies are constantly under siege by cancer cells. It's nothing unusual because, under normal circumstances, these harmful cells never get a chance to take hold and cause any real damage because a well-functioning immune system prevents this from occurring. It's when the immune system becomes compromised in some way, or the assault from cancer-promoting forces too great, that problems emerge.

The way it's supposed to work is like this: a healthy, aerobic cellular system metabolizes both oxygen and glucose from food, producing ATP that serves as the energy store for cells to perform their various functions. In the process, ATP production releases carbon dioxide that's used by the body to extract oxygen from hemoglobin, the red blood cells responsible for transporting oxygen from the lungs to the cells. All the while the immune system keeps everything in check and prevents malignant cells—cells that aren't doing their job—from taking over and wreaking havoc on the body.

The way it's *not* supposed to work, and the reason why some people end up developing full-blown "cancer" in the conventional sense, is that cancer cells become so great in number that they start siphoning off glucose and using it for their own proliferation. Healthy cells are consequently deprived of this much-needed blood sugar, leading to a loss of homeostasis and an overtaking of the body by this army of increasingly virulent cancer cells, a process that, if left unchecked, can lead to *systemic* (i.e., much more difficult to treat) cancer of the entire body.

This means that glucose, the very substance that would otherwise be beneficial to a well-functioning cellular system, becomes the body's *worst nightmare* when cancer cells are in charge. Cancer cells begin to use glucose as their own food, excreting lactic acid back into the bloodstream where it is sent to the liver and converted back into glucose, providing even more food for cancer cells.

It's a vicious cycle that can only be broken with the right interventions, *none* of which include the administration of chemotherapy or radiation treatments. Again, these conventional methods only make the problem *worse* by not only generating more cancer cells, but also converting those that already exist into cancer *stem* cells, which by their very nature act as manufacturers of new cancer cells.[2]

So if healthy cells operate aerobically to metabolize oxygen and glucose as a means to generate ATP, the lifeblood of the body, then it's only logical that cancer cells operate *anaerobically*. The anaerobic nature of cancer cells is such that very little oxygen is metabolized, resulting in very little ATP being produced. Anaerobic cells are also incapable of producing carbon dioxide as a byproduct of ATP production, which means they can't pull oxygen out of hemoglobin.

This weakness creates a major energy deficiency throughout the body and inhibits the body from producing protective antioxidant enzymes like superoxide dismutase, glutathione peroxidase, catalase, and reductase. It also creates a systemic lack of oxygen for not only healthy cells but also the cancer cells themselves, which in turn begin to form their own new blood vessels, a process known as angiogenesis, just to get the oxygen and sugar they need to survive.

Because of their anaerobic nature, cancer cells have to initiate angiogenesis for their own survival. It's a process that further deprives healthy areas of the body of the oxygen and glucose *they* need to produce energy and stay alive, and cancer cells exert constant leeching of energy on healthy cells as they grow and spread.

Dr. David Gregg explains how the process works with succinct clarity: "Cancer does not cause cells to turn anaerobic, but rather it is stabilized anaerobic respiration that is the single cause (or essential requirement) that turns the normal cells that depend on aerobic respiration into cancer cells." He adds concerning the angiogenic activity of cancer cells:

> Normal cells in the oxygen deficient environment of the anaerobic tumor cells may be creating the new blood vessels, not the cancer cells. . . . It is well known that in order for tumors to grow they must form new blood vessels to supply the increased tumor size. . . . Thus, anaerobic metabolism is not just a secondary consequence of cancer; it is a requirement for cancer to grow.

In other words, it would be impossible for cancer cells to spur the angiogenic process of new blood vessel formation, which is essential to their very survival, if they weren't anaerobically stunted in the first place. The fact that cancer cells are inherently *weaker* than healthy cells precludes their hostile takeover and restructuring of cellular metabolism.

So where does cancer actually begin? Paul Gerhardt Seeger, a prominent scientific researcher who was twice nominated for the Nobel Prize, theorized in the 1930s that ground zero is the cytoplasm of the cell: this mass of gel-like fluid, which is where the cell's mitochondria, or energy-producing "engine," is located, acts as a platform for the conversion of healthy cells into cancer cells.

When the cell's normal "respiratory chain," as he called it, becomes blocked, whether due to enzymatic failure or some other factor that leads to a breakdown in the process, aerobic cells turn into anaerobic cells. He successfully proved this theory in an experiment where he introduced a chemical into a healthy cell culture, which within a matter of *days* transformed into an unhealthy cell one.[3]

Seeger's colleague, Otto Warburg, held a similar view of cancer. He correctly theorized that cancer cells generate energy nonoxidatively, altering the pathways of normal cellular metabolism and consequently generating cancer "masses," or what we would call tumors, that are the direct result of damaged cell respiration.

In his 1966 paper entitled "The Prime Cause and Prevention of Cancer," Warburg breaks down in fervent detail how cancer is essentially the replacement of this normal respiration process in healthy cells with the "fermentation of sugar" in unhealthy ones.[4] This change, which he dubbed "respiration injury," is now regarded as the most fundamental metabolic alteration responsible for generating malignant cancer cells.

At the same time, Seeger demonstrated that these respiration injuries can be fully *reversed*, leading to a *restoration process* whereby anaerobic (cancerous) cells are converted back into aerobic (healthy) cells. He even pinpointed the precise enzyme that, when inactivated or destroyed, precipitates the initial formation of cancer cells.

"In 1938 Paul Seeger discovered that cancer results from the inactivation or destruction of the most important enzyme of the respiratory chain, cytochrome oxidase, or more specifically, cytochrome a/a3," explains Professor Serge Jurasunas, M.D., in a scientific paper he published on the subject.

Cytochrome a/a3, it turns out, is *by far* the most important mitochondrial respiratory enzyme because it's responsible for processing in excess of 90 percent of the oxygen consumed by the body. Without this "biological catalyst," the mitochondria would have no way of receiving this oxygen; hence, this is why a lack of fully functioning cytochrome a/a3 is associated with major disruptions in the cellular respiratory chain. Jurasunas states:

> Paul Seeger proved in his 310 scientific works of basic research that the results of thousands of carefully conducted electrochemical experiments and hundreds of histological experiments confirmed his early research . . . concerning the inactivation and destruction of cytochrome a/a3 (cytochrome oxidase) as a factor that initiates

cancer. He was able to prove that oxygen transported by erythro-cytes (red blood cells) can only be utilized in the mitochondria if certain respiratory enzymes (cytochrome oxidases) are present.[5]

The solutions that Seeger and his protégés came up with to address the issue of disrupted cellular respiration are the subject matter of later chapters. But I wanted to lay the initial groundwork for what cancer is and how it forms at the cellular level so you have a better understanding of the true nature of this disease as we move forward together on this important journey.

CANCER IS A MODERN DISEASE

As far as the history of cancer itself goes, the earliest evidence we have of its existence dates back to only about the 17th century. Historical records and actual mummified remains prior to this time point to cancer being virtually *nonexistent,* or at the very least exceptionally rare. The reason for this, historians agree, is that ancient civilizations ate cleaner food and weren't exposed to the same toxic chemicals and pollution as we are today in the post-industrial age.

Researchers from the U.K. took a closer look at the issue in 2010, poring through classical literature, the fossil record, and actual mummified bodies to look for any evidence of cancer prior to roughly 200 years ago. They examined tissue samples from hundreds of Egyptian mummies and found only *one* that showed even the possibility of cancer, leading one of the study's lead investigators, Michael Zimmerman, a visiting professor at Manchester University, to make the following admission: "In an ancient society lacking surgical intervention, evidence of cancer should remain in all cases. The virtual absence of malignancies in mummies must be interpreted as indicating their rarity in antiquity, indicating that cancer-causing factors are limited to societies affected by modern industrialization."

As to whether cancer has always been with us as an inevitable fate for some, or if it's a product of something we're doing *wrong* in the modern age, Professor Rosalie David, who presented the study's findings before a meeting of oncologists, stated:

> There is nothing in the natural environment that can cause cancer. So it has to be a man-made disease, down to pollution and changes to our diet and lifestyle. . . . We can make very clear statements on the cancer rates in societies because we have a full overview. We have looked at millennia, not one hundred years, and have masses of data.
>
> Yet again extensive ancient Egyptian data, along with other data from across the millennia, has given modern society a clear message—cancer is man-made and something that we can and should address.[6]

If cancer has really been around since the beginning of time as the American Cancer Society and other prominent cancer groups claim, then why do we see little, if any, evidence of its existence prior to the industrial revolution? What was once a practically nonexistent disease is now the *second-leading* killer in developed countries, and the *number-one* killer in "underdeveloped" countries; this includes developing countries as well.

The National Cancer Institute estimates that 1,685,210 new cases of cancer will be diagnosed in the United States in 2016. This translates to about 4,617 new cases of cancer every day, 192 new cases of cancer every hour, and more than 3 new cases of cancer *every minute.*

The NCI also estimates that in 2016, 595,690 people will *die* from cancer—or more realistically, from cancer *treatments* like chemotherapy and radiation. This translates to 1,632 cancer deaths every single day in 2016, 68 deaths from cancer every hour, and more than 1 cancer death every minute. Nearly 10 percent of the 1,685,210 new people afflicted by cancer ever year are children 19 years of age or younger. And more than 3 percent of the 595,690 who die are children, most of whom suffered from cancers of the brain, central nervous system, and blood.

Cancer is so common in the modern age that it is now the leading cause of death worldwide, claiming the lives of some 8.2 million people per year, according to World Health Organization (WHO) data from 2012. Globally speaking, one out of every eight deaths that occurs, or 12.5 percent, is attributable to cancer. This figure is even worse in the U.S., with one in *four* deaths the result of cancer.

Upwards of 14 million new cases of cancer will be diagnosed next year, and this number is expected to nearly double to 22 million cases per year by the time we reach 2036. And try this little factoid on for size: roughly 40 percent of the general population will be diagnosed with cancer at some point throughout their lives—nearly one out of every two people![7]

If you're married, this means that statistically, either you or your spouse will someday develop cancer. If you're a woman, it will probably be some form of breast cancer. If you're a man, it very well could manifest as prostate cancer. I'm not trying to scare you with this, but rather give you some perspective as to just how prolific this nefarious disease has become.

"A contemporary woman's risk of breast cancer is 54% greater than was her mother's at the same age among blacks and 41% greater among whites," reported a 1999 study published in the journal *Annual Review of Public Health*.[8] "Men today have about a three- to four-fold risk of being diagnosed with prostate cancer compared with their fathers."

And this is relatively old data; the situation has gotten progressively *worse* over the past several decades. In the year 2000, the total number of new breast cancer cases in the U.S. was 182,800.[9] Fast-forward 16 years and this number is expected to be 246,660 in 2016, an increase of about 35 percent.

"During the past half-century, the lifetime risk of breast cancer more than tripled in the United States," reports the group Breast Cancer Action. "In the 1940s, a woman's lifetime risk of breast cancer was one in 22. In 2004, it was one in seven. In 2007, it decreased to one in eight."[10]

So while there have been a few slight dips over the years in the overall incidence rate of breast cancer, making for some convenient sound-bites to show that we're "winning" the war on breast cancer, the truth is that general trends tell a much different story. And we see the same thing with prostate cancer in men, and with many other forms of cancer in both men and women.

Believe it or not, prostate cancer is actually the most commonly diagnosed form of cancer besides skin cancer in the U.S. Nearly a quarter-million American men were diagnosed with it in 2012, and more than 28,000 died from it that same year.[11]

Similar trends are apparent with cancers of the lungs, colon, rectum, bladder, skin, thyroid, kidney, pelvis, pancreas, and blood. They're *all* increasing steadily, some more than others and admittedly with dips, but increasing nonetheless. And the burden on society to provide care and treatment for all these patients is tremendous.

CANCER IS THE BIGGEST FINANCIAL DRAIN ON SOCIETY

Unless you or a loved has undergone conventional treatment for cancer, you likely aren't aware of the astronomical costs associated with these procedures. Estimates compiled by *DrugWatch* put the annual cost of treating cancer at nearly $1 *trillion*, topping that of traffic accidents and diabetes *combined*. The aggregate costs associated with cancer treatment exceed even that of heart disease, the number-one killer in the U.S.

Per patient, cancer treatment now exceeds $200,000 per year, up more than 50 percent from about $139,000 per year in 2005. Some of the newest cancer drugs are even more expensive than this: an FDA-approved skin cancer treatment manufactured by Bristol-Myers Squibb that's only about 60 percent effective at shrinking—but not necessarily curing—tumors costs $141,000 per three months, and roughly $256,000 annually.

The American Institute of Cancer Research (AICR) says that cancer is, hands down, the most costly disease to treat. Its costs aren't just monetary in terms of payment for treatments, but also socially in terms of lost life and productivity. Here's how *DrugWatch* breaks it all down: "The biggest financial impact (of cancer) is in terms of loss of life and productivity, in which cancer accounts for 1.5 percent of global gross domestic products (GDP) losses. The AICR estimates Americans lost 83 million years of healthy life because of cancer deaths and disabilities in 2008."[12]

In the U.S., the total cost of treating cancer in 2010 totaled $124.5 billion. A 2011 study published in the *Journal of the National Cancer Institute* projects that by the year 2020, this cost will jump to $157.7 billion, an increase of 27 percent. More people developing cancer is partially to blame for this, but so are escalating prices for conventional drug-based treatments.[13]

Research compiled by the National Bureau of Economic Research found that anticancer drugs have increased in price by about 10 percent *every single year* since 1995, with no end in sight. Based on current price schedules, this amounts to increases of about $8,500 annually, after adjusting for inflation and survival benefits.[14]

Mind you, these are treatments that almost *never* actually cure cancer. In some cases, they may help extend a patient's life by a few extra months or perhaps a year or two. But we're talking about year-after-year *survival* rates, in which patients with cancer more often than not still have cancer but are just "managing" it with expensive drugs. And this management process is draining the financial coffers of our nation at an alarming rate, all the while leaving cancer patients without any real hope of truly overcoming their cancers: "When calculating the average cost for one extra year of life, the researchers determined patients and insurers paid $54,100 in 1995. The price for one year of life increased to $139,100 in 2005 and $207,000 in 2013," *DrugWatch* explains.

These are just the costs for treatment itself; realistically, a cancer patient and his or her family incur added costs from missed work, transportation, special meals, child care, advanced equipment, clothing, and more. And with insurance companies increasingly reluctant to cover the latest high-dollar treatment offerings, many cancer patients and their families have to resort to consulting lawyers to try to recoup their losses.

The financial toll in terms of lost productivity is also enormous. A 2014 study published in the *International Journal of Cancer* estimated that in Europe alone, the annual cost to society from lives lost to cancer is about $84 billion. Deaths associated with breast cancer account for $7.84 billion of this figure.[15] I say "associated" here because, as I mentioned earlier, many deaths due to cancer are actually deaths caused by cancer *treatment*. So after paying tens, or even *hundreds*, of thousands of dollars in an attempt to get better, many cancer patients end up dying from the very regimens they thought would heal them, resulting in even more costs to the patient's family and society at large.

To call this spinning hamster wheel of false hope and failure a financial disaster of unsustainable proportions barely scratches the surface. It's painfully ironic that a system claiming to address malignancies of the cellular system is the biggest social and financial malignancy of the modern world.

While the cogs that make up the wheel of conventional cancer care are admittedly complex—the financial costs, the societal costs, and the physical costs of treatment among them—there's just no denying the simple fact that what we're doing *just isn't working*. Cancer rates are skyrocketing despite more money than ever before being shoveled into the coffers of the cancer industry. Something has to change, and fast, in order to avoid the inevitable financial collapse that will result if we continue along the course of business as usual. It's time to suck up our pride, admit that the current system is broken, and work toward developing *real* solutions to cancer that aren't proprietary, not to mention prohibitively costly.

Truth be told, conventional cancer treatments are already so out of reach for the average American that even with excellent insurance coverage, a cancer diagnosis can mean absolute financial ruin; this is even true for folks in the upper middle class of the socioeconomic stratum. Just imagine what it's like for people living in underdeveloped and developing countries of the world, where cancer rates are currently skyrocketing higher than anywhere else on the planet.

Cancer drugs are also much more costly in the U.S. than they are in many other places due to monopolistic pricing schemes that benefit the drug industry at the expense of patients. A common leukemia drug known as Gleevac, for instance, costs about $70,000 to administer here in the states. In India, the exact same drug costs a mere $2,500.[16]

Even closer to home, many of the exact same cancer drugs sold for a premium here in the U.S. are available in Canada for a fraction of the cost. Popular breast cancer drugs like tamoxifen are one example of this, costing in some cases *one-tenth* of what they cost in the U.S.,[17] simply due to the fact that drug companies are getting away with robbing Americans blind—thanks to a Congress that refuses to negotiate on behalf of the people for whom it's supposed to be working.

"Existing regulations are what drive up the prices and prevent competition," writes Logan Albright for FreedomWorks, pointing out that the FDA restricts the import of cheaper, equivalent drugs from other countries because doing so not only ensures that the FDA will continue to receive its new drug application user fees, but also that its pharmaceutical "clients" remain protected from outside competition. "Making it easier and cheaper to bring drugs to market, as well as allowing the importation of safe medicines from other countries would increase supply and lower costs, greatly hampering the ability of even the most ruthless businessman to corner the market on saving lives."[18]

I'm in full agreement, except I would advocate for taking things a step further and opening up the market to other treatment modalities for cancer, many of which I'll cover in later chapters. The only way to end this monopolistic drug system and make available to the public real healing solutions at the lowest possible cost is to bring back real competition in medicine.

CHAPTER 6

CANCER CAUSES . . .
IS CANCER GENETIC?

So what *actually* causes cancer? I briefly touched on this earlier when I highlighted some of the metabolic abnormalities that cause cancer cells to spring out of healthy cells and take hold in the form of cancerous tumors. But how are these abnormalities triggered in the first place—and more importantly, what, if any, outside influences help push the body over the edge into cancer territory?

The official position of the National Cancer Institute is that cancer is purely a genetic disease. The government agency maintains that cancer is caused by certain genetic changes that alter the way cells divide, resulting in various mutations and tumor growths. Our ancestry and the "faulty" genes that were passed down to us by our parents and grandparents, the NCI also claims, are major determining factors in whether or not we as individuals will develop cancer at some point in our lives.

Whether inherited or somatic (acquired throughout the course of one's life), genetic changes are said to be the linchpin in the birth and proliferation of cancer, and there's not much the average person can do to thwart the process besides avoiding cigarettes and staying out of the sun. You read that right: the NCI sees our premier source of light and the primary means by which our bodies produce vitamin D to be a significant threat to our genome.

This oft-repeated narrative that genetic "defects" are somehow responsible for causing cancer has pervaded the collective consciousness, so much so that many people now throw caution to the wind and just live however they wish because they've been inadvertently programmed to say "*everything* causes cancer." I've heard this type of statement on many occasions from people who don't know the first thing about the importance of diet and lifestyle in relation to cancer, and I'm sure you have as well.

It's a defeatist mind-set predicated on the notion that cancer can't actually be prevented with any sort of habitual routine of healthy living, only *possibly* avoided through mostly chance—and this is a matter of being lucky enough to have been born with "good" genes. Nothing could be more painfully misguided when it comes to understanding the world's leading killer, but this is how many people think because it's what their doctors tell them and it's what federal agencies like the NCI claim represents a proper "scientific" understanding of the nature of cancer.

Truth be told, genetic abnormalities are just a *symptom* of cancer, not the cause. And the vast majority of them aren't hereditary, but rather somatically corporeal, which simply means they're brought about as a result of external influences like poor diet and toxic exposure. Only about *5 percent* of all cancers are attributable to one's ancestry.[1] The rest are a product of one's *environment*.

CANCER ISN'T GENETIC; IT'S THE RESULT OF IMMUNE FAILURE

Cancer, in essence, can be summed up as a *failure of the immune system* to eradicate abnormal cells before they take root and become full-blown cancer. Our bodies are literally teeming with cancer cells to the tune of hundreds of thousands of new ones daily, which isn't anything out of the ordinary when the immune system is functioning optimally. When it's not, that's when problems arise.

"Our immune system's job is to get rid of those cells—*if* your immune system is perfect, if you don't have a virus that it's already trying to fight, if you don't have too much chemical or other stuff going on in your body," Dr. Bita Badakhshan, M.D., an integrative medicine physician at the Center for New Medicine in Irvine, California, explained to me during an interview for *The Truth About Cancer: A Global Quest.* "If you do," she told me plainly, "then [these malignant cells] keep growing and growing and increasing in number, and then you get a tumor."

It's really as simple as that. When a healthy cell gets out of line and fails to follow through with apoptosis, a normal process of programmed cell death, the immune system is designed to go after it and destroy it. When the immune system is compromised in some way, cancer cells are given an "in" to continue reproducing forever until they eventually destroy the body.

Dr. Badakhshan, who started off her career as a conventional doctor, says many of the patients she sees at the Center for New Medicine suffer from immune suppression caused by persistent viruses: things like HPV (human papillomavirus), herpes, mono (mononucleosis) and Epstein-Barr. Lyme disease and parasites, she says, are also common predicators of cancer, and conditions she's observed countless times throughout her practice in conjunction with cancer diagnoses. "What does the parasite do to your body? It suppresses the immune system," she warns. "There are doctors who believe people develop cancer because of the parasite, some believe candida, some fungus and yeast—I believe everything has to do with that."

Reiterating much of what I covered in the last chapter, Dr. Badakhshan subscribes to the metabolic theory of cancer, upholding that the true cause of this disease is rooted in mitochondrial dysfunction stemming from inadequate oxygen delivery to healthy cells. The resulting lack of ATP production combined with immune shutdown creates the perfect environment for cancer to thrive.

Dr. Aleksandra Niedzwiecki, Ph.D., director of research at the Dr. Rath Research Institute in Santa Clara, California, puts it like this: "Cancer is a process that occurs in our body all the time. As we are sitting and talking, there are cancer cells that are constantly created in our body. They do not always lead to the development of cancer because our immune system finds them as abnormal cells and eliminates them."

When the immune system is damaged, these cancer cells, which divide "indefinitely," start spreading, or metastasizing, and invading other organs. And it's this metastasizing action that kills the vast majority of cancer patients—that and the destructive treatments many scared and desperate cancer patients subject themselves to in the name of science-based medicine.

PESTICIDES, ANTIBIOTICS, GROWTH HORMONES, AND POLLUTION: THE ENVIRONMENTAL EFFECT

One of the things I learned about cancer that really shocked me was the fact that most cancer deaths aren't attributable to the primary cancer itself, but to cancer metastasis: when cancer spreads far and wide throughout the body and makes its home in vital organs and other important areas. By the time cancer reaches this level, which can take five years, ten years, or even longer, it's already too late.

This is why prevention, or at the very least *early detection*, is so important in the fight against cancer. Knowing the factors and influences that contribute to the formation of cancer is the key to prevention, so what exactly are these? One major grouping is environmental toxins: things like crop pesticides and herbicides, antibiotic drugs, artificial growth hormones, and other forms of pollution that obstruct oxygen uptake and damage immunity.

The viruses, bacteria, fungi, and yeast that Dr. Badakhshan spoke about as contributing factors to cancer are only as detrimental as the bodies they invade allow them to be. Again, immune failure is at the root of what allows cancer cells to flourish and spread, and more often than not this destruction of natural immunity is a product of toxic overload.

After years of beckoning from the public and public interest groups to spearhead an investigation into the environmental contributors to cancer, the President's Cancer Panel compiled a report in 2009 declaring that the true burden of environmentally induced cancer "has been grossly underestimated. . . . With nearly 80,000 chemicals on the market in the United States, many of which are used by millions of Americans in their daily lives and are un- or understudied and largely unregulated, exposure to potential environmental carcinogens is widespread."

With candid urgency in its petition to the president, the panel added:

> The American people—even before they are born—are bombarded continually with myriad combinations of these dangerous exposures. The Panel urges you most strongly to use the power of your office to remove the carcinogens and other toxins from our food, water, and air that needlessly increase the health care costs, cripple our Nation's productivity, and devastate American lives.[2]

Dr. Rob Verkerk, Ph.D., executive director of the Alliance for Natural Health International, offers further insights into this major problem, noting that the average city dweller is exposed to upwards of 20,000 industrial chemicals *every single day*. Many of these chemicals are known carcinogens, and the vast majority of them emerged after the World War II as adjuncts to natural compounds that couldn't be patented, and thus weren't profitable to the chemical industry barons. "After the war, we saw this massive evolution both in terms of agrochemicals and pharmaceuticals of patented molecules that became the business model," he told me during a recent interview.

The emergence of this newfound chemical industry cracked open a Pandora's box of destruction, unleashing a host of cancer-causing agents into the world that over at least the past half century have contributed in a significant way to the major uptick in cancer rates that we see all around the world in nearly every statistical model. To help you grasp the scope of this, I'd like to break down some of the worst offenders that many of us are exposed to on a daily basis:

1) CROP CHEMICALS

Ever since the fall of mankind, the earth hasn't exactly been the most hospitable to human survival endeavors like farming and agriculture. Weeds and pests are part of the "curse," so to speak, and civilizations throughout history have attempted to thwart their deleterious effects with pesticides, herbicides, and insecticides. Prior to the industrial revolution, such interventions were mostly natural. Ancient Sumerians, for instance, used sulfur to control insects and mites, while Greco-Romans used "smokes" to fight mildew and blight. Cultivators burned materials like straw, hedge clippings, and even animal dung to create a thick smoke, which would then be blown into the wind across a field or orchard. It was also common to use plant extracts like bitter lupin and wild cucumber to deter insects.[3]

Many plants contain their own natural pest deterrents, and some cultures have extracted and concentrate these for use in the crop fields. Pyrethrum, a derivative of Pyrethrum daisies (*Chrysanthemum cinerariaefolium*), is a broad-spectrum botanical insecticide that's been in use for more than 2,000 years. A Bordeaux mixture of copper sulfate and lime is another natural solution that's long been used to treat fungal diseases on crops.

During the mid-20th century, many of the organic and inorganic substances that had been in use forever were replaced with chemical by-products of coal and oil production, the boon sectors of the industrial revolution. Synthetic pesticides gained a strong footing during this time, supplanting nearly all other methods of crop management—but not without a price. The introduction of early synthetics like nitrophenols, chlorophenols, creosate, naphthalene, and other petroleum-derived substances for fungal infections and insect pests, as well as ammonium sulfate and sodium arsenate for weeds, *seemed* like a logical solution to the nation's agricultural woes. But these chemicals would prove detrimental to environmental and human health.

Indiscriminate use of these first-generation crop chemicals throughout the earlier part of the 20th century would lead to the introduction of second- and even third-generation crop chemicals during the latter part of the century. During the 1970s and 1980s, a weed killer known as glyphosate would emerge, as would a host of other pesticides like *Bacillus thuringiensis* (Bt) and pyrethroids, the latter of which is a synthetic knock-off of natural Pyrethrum.

We also saw the introduction of herbicides from the "imi" (i.e., imidazolinone), "fop" (i.e. aryloxyphenoxypropionate), and "dim" (i.e., cyclohexanediones) families; insecticides like avermectins and benzoylureas; and fungicides like pyrimidine, imidazole, and triazole, all of which work somewhat well *initially*, but cause other problems over time.

"As many of the agrochemicals introduced at this time had a single mode of action, thus making them more selective, problems with resistance occurred," says John Unsworth of the International Union of Pure and Applied Chemistry. Resistance is something that only gets worse, not better, as a result of chemical-intensive crop management practices. This is why the chemical industry resorted to introducing genetically modified, or GMO, crops in the mid-1990s as a solution to the problem it created with synthetic pesticides.[4]

But widespread monocropping and layer after layer of pesticides have not only *not* solved the problem of pests and weeds; they've also done a number on public health. The Pesticide Action Network of North America has been tracking the progression of chronic disease in conjunction with crop chemical use over many decades, and the data is sobering. "Chemicals can trigger cancer in a variety of ways, including disrupting hormones, damaging DNA, inflaming tissues and turning genes on or off. Many pesticides are 'known or probable' carcinogens and, as the President's Panel notes, exposure to these chemicals is widespread."[5]

Children are most affected by these chemicals, as are expectant mothers who inadvertently expose their unborn children to chemicals in utero. Farm workers exposed to pesticides on a regular basis have it pretty bad as well, reporting significantly higher rates of prostate (in men), ovarian (in women), and skin cancers.

Crop chemicals are intensely pervasive, meaning they bioaccumulate in the environment and human tissue. Glyphosate, which is sold under the Monsanto-owned brand Roundup, is now the world's most extensively used crop chemical, and a recent study published in the journal *Environmental Toxicology Chemistry* found that it is now present at detectable levels in up to 75 percent of air and rain samples.[6] Glyphosate, by the way, was originally developed in 1964 as a chelator of minerals, trace minerals, and especially magnesium. It pulls these minerals from the soils on which it's sprayed, as well as from the bodies of people who've been exposed to it. It's a nasty chemical, and these days it's *everywhere*, much to the detriment of current and future generations.

The effect that glyphosate and other crop chemicals have on magnesium levels in the body is particularly concerning as magnesium is essential for more than 300 functions of the body. Magnesium deficiency is a major risk factor for cancer because this essential mineral is used by the cells for ATP production and energy generation.

"We have sprayed pesticides . . . throughout our shared environment," laments biologist and cancer survivor Sandra Steingraber, whose statements on cancer and pesticides are included in the President's Cancer Panel report. "They are now in amniotic fluid. They're in our blood. They're in our urine. They're in our exhaled breath. They are in mothers' milk . . . What is the burden of cancer that we can attribute to this use of poisons in our agricultural system? . . . We won't really know the answer until we do the other experiment—which is to take the poisons out of our food chain, embrace a different kind of agriculture, and see what happens."[7]

2) GENETICALLY MODIFIED ORGANISMS (GMOS)

The chemical toxicity component of modern agriculture is just one part of the problem; the other is transgenic crop species. Despite their official status as "food," GMOs are essentially drugs that have been sneaked into the food supply without consent, with mounds of independent research exposing them as a health disaster.

The FDA has never required proper safety testing for GMOs because it agrees with the chemical industry that GMOs are substantially equivalent to non-GMOs—except when it comes to patent protection, of course. Yet we see in independent tests that long-term GMO consumption is associated with a number of serious health conditions.

> Several animal studies indicate serious health risks associated with GM food consumption including infertility, immune dysregulation, accelerated aging, dysregulation of genes associated with cholesterol synthesis, insulin regulation, cell signaling, and protein formation, and changes in the liver, kidney, spleen and gastrointestinal system," reports the American Academy of Environmental Medicine (AAEM).[8]

GMOs that manufacture their own internal pesticides are also high risk, according to Jeffrey M. Smith, GMO expert, filmmaker, researcher, lecturer, and head of the Institute for Responsible Technology. He explained to me during a recent interview that *Bacillus thuringiensis* that's engineered into corn alters gut bacteria and increases one's risk of developing cancer. "If the Bt gene transfers to gut bacteria and continues to function it can convert our intestinal flora into living pesticide factories producing Bt toxin 24/7 which might poke holes along the cell walls causing inflammation and all sorts of gastrointestinal disorders, possibly creating leaky gut, which is also linked to cancer," Smith told me in a 2014 interview.

The biotechnology industry has spent vast amounts of money and time defending GMOs as a necessary component to ending world hunger. But like its claims about their safety, the idea that GMOs are more efficient and produce higher yields than traditional foods is a lie, which is why groups like the AAEM are calling for an immediate moratorium on their cultivation and use in the food supply.

3) ENVIRONMENTAL TOXINS
You can't always see them, but environmental pollutants are everywhere and many of them are carcinogenic. They're obvious when they're billowing out of a smokestack or puffing out of an exhaust pipe, but some of the worst ones are hiding unseen in soil and water, and even in foods that you probably eat on a regular basis. Some are naturally occurring and some are industrial waste by-products; as is the case with arsenic, some are *both*. The National Cancer Institute lists the following toxins as being the most likely environmental carcinogens that affect human health:

Aflatoxins (a type of mycotoxic fungi that occurs on some food crops), aristolochic acid (present in some plants), arsenic (often released from mining and metal smelting), asbestos (in old buildings), benzene (a chemical and pharmaceutical solvent), benzidine (in some clothing dyes), beryllium (a natural metal), 1,3-butadiene (used to produce synthetic rubber), cadmium (a natural element), coal tar and coal-tar pitch, coke-oven emissions, crystalline silica (a respirable size), erionite (found in zeolite rock), ethylene oxide (a chemical in antifreeze), formaldehyde (a chemical often used in building materials), hexavalent chromium compounds, mineral oils, nickel compounds, radon (a radioactive gas released from the earth), secondhand cigarette smoke, soot, sulfuric acid, thorium (a radioactive metal), vinyl chloride (used to make PVC plastic), and wood dust.[9]

A number of other substances that I believe should be on this list as well include:

- *Triclosan*, an antibacterial chemical often used in hand soaps
- *Perfluorooctanoic acid* (PFOA), a chemical used in Teflon and other nonstick cookware
- *Volatile organic compounds* (VOCs), a class of highly toxic chemical used in carpeting. VOCs generate formaldehyde, benzene, and other cancer-causing chemicals like acetaldehyde, toluene, and perchloroethylene
- *Parabens*, a type of cancer-causing chemical used in shampoos and perfumes
- *Alkyloamides*, a class of chemicals used to emulsify hand lotions and soaps
- *Aluminum*, a toxic metal added to antiperspirant deodorants
- *Oxybenzone*, a cancer-causing chemical added to many commercial sunscreens
- *Sodium polyacrylate* (SAP), a chemical agent used in disposable diapers

And we can't forget about the various other mycotoxins lurking out there like citrinin, fumonisin B1 and B2, ochratoxin A, ergot alkaloid, zearalenone, and trichothecenes. These names might not mean all that much to you, but each of these microfungi metabolites, many of which are hiding in food, pose a serious threat to your health.

Conventional corn is loaded with fumonisins, which are linked to kidney and liver damage, defects of the brain and spinal cord (in human embryos), and esophageal cancer. Trichothecenes, a class of fungi that grows on cereal grains, inhibit protein synthesis and interfere with cell function: think cancer.[10]

4) VACCINES

These "miracles" of public health are loaded with chemical preservatives and adjuvants that are known carcinogens, not to mention live viruses that, in many cases, compromise and weaken immunity. Additives like formaldehyde (rat poison), aluminum, and mercury (thimerosal) are some of the worst offenders you'll find in vaccines, as are petroleum-based food colorings, acetone (a flammable solvent), aborted human fetal cells, and ammonium.[11]

Both the Environmental Protection Agency and the World Health Organization's International Agency for Research on Cancer (IARC) classify formaldehyde as a cancer-causing substance. Studies have also shown that formaldehyde is a DNA adduct, meaning it acts as a type of precursor in the birthing of new cancer cells, basically pushing the body toward a full-blown cancer diagnosis at some point in the future.[12]

Concerns about the safety of mercury, commonly listed on vaccine package inserts as thimerosal, have predicated its removal from many of the vaccines on the CDC schedule. But contrary to what you may have heard, it's still used in the production of multidose vials of influenza vaccine, as well as in vaccines for diphtheria, meningitis, and tetanus.

The link between mercury and autism is well established, with the overall neurotoxicity of this metal a significant factor in speech disorders and other neurodevelopmental delays in children. Studies have also linked mercury to tumors of the kidneys, lungs, and central nervous system.[13]

Aluminum is another biggie in vaccines, and for what purpose is anyone's guess. Aluminum salts like aluminum hydroxide are supposed to amplify the immune response provoked by the vaccine antigens themselves, but research shows that this "soft" metal is a major factor in macrophagic myofasciitis, or MMF, as well as autism.

And then there's the controversial SV40 virus, which was originally extracted from rhesus monkey kidney cells back in the 1950s to produce the first vaccine for polio. Though it was supposed to have been phased out decades ago, SV40 was reportedly added to vaccines given to children until at least the 1990s.

The infamous Salk vaccine for polio, which contained SV40, was shown in a study published in the *New England Journal of Medicine* to increase the risk of brain tumors by about 1,300 percent. The virus has also been detected in association with osteogenic sarcomas and human mesotheliomas.

5) MOBILE PHONES AND EMFS

If it's not pressed up against your thigh at this very moment, it's probably in your hand or glued to your ear. I'm talking about your mobile phone, the 24/7 companion that, for most people, never leaves their side except at night while they sleep—and even then it's usually plugged in and charging just a few inches away from their heads.

All this contact with these convenient devices is problematic because they're constantly emitting electromagnetic radiation that the IARC says is "possibly" carcinogenic to humans.[14] Despite their classification as low-powered radio-frequency transmitters, mobile phones act similarly to microwave ovens in the way they emit radiation, heating up water molecules with which they come into contact.

A mobile phone pressed directly against your head while it's sending and receiving frequency and data will inadvertently "cook" your brain cells, since this tissue is composed primarily of water. The long-term effects of this are poorly understood, but common sense dictates that cooking brain tissue on a regular basis is a recipe for cancer, particularly cancer of the brain.

Even when mobile phone radiation isn't cooking cell tissue, it still damages the way brain cells function, according to a 2011 study conducted by researchers at the National Institutes of Health. These same radio-frequency (RF) waves from mobile phones generate "stress" proteins in human cells, says Martin Blank, Ph.D., who lectures on physiology and cellular biophysics at Columbia University in New York.[15]

A German study published in the *Journal of Negative Results in BioMedicine* in 2015 concluded that, based on a review of the published science, there exists "some evidence to suggest a connection between heavy mobile phone use and increased risk for brain tumor occurrence, especially for gliomas."[16]

6) FLUORIDE

They say it prevents tooth decay, but fluoride, which is added to many municipal water supplies, is a known mutagen. The National Toxicology Program has concluded based on "the preponderance of evidence" that fluoride chemicals are mutagenic, meaning they inflict the type of genetic damage that later on down the road can trigger the formation of cancer.[17]

Contrary to what you were probably told all your life, fluoride isn't safe, even at the supposedly "low" doses that are laced into public water supplies. This is because fluoride is bioaccumulative, meaning it builds up over time into so-called "microenvironments" like the brain, bones, and vital organs. According to the Fluoride Action Network, at least seven studies published over the last 30 years have found evidence of genetic damage in conjunction with fluoride exposure. One of these, published in 2006 in the journal *Cancer, Causes & Control,* made the following assessment with regards to bone cancer in young boys:

> We observed that for males diagnosed before the age of 20 years, fluoride levels in drinking water during growth was associated with an increased risk of osteosarcoma, demonstrating a peak in the odds ratio from 6 to 8 years of age. All of our models were remarkably robust in showing this effect, which coincides with the mid-childhood growth spurt."[18]

This would make sense as fluoride competes with iodine, a *beneficial* mineral, for residency in cell tissue. Fluoride actually supplants iodine in the thyroid gland, a contributing factor to thyroid cancer. Fluoride exposure has also been linked to cancers of the skin, bladder, and lungs.[19]

7) PLASTICS

There's really nothing good to say about plastic in general, as this petroleum derivative isn't exactly doing our bodies or the environment any favors. But some forms of plastic are worse than others, lending to a higher likelihood of hormonal changes and possible cancers as a result of long-term exposure.

Many of the chemicals that are added to plastics to make them flexible, durable, and fit for various other functions are highly toxic; a great number of them are also carcinogenic. One of the most well known is bisphenol-A, or BPA, a plasticizing chemical used in water bottles that was shown in a 2014 study to predispose rats to breast cancer.[20]

Like fluoride, BPA appears to be mutagenic in the way that it alters genetic expression, potentially leading to cancer. And there are many other plastics chemicals with similar cancer-causing propensity:[21]

- Phthalates like diethylhexyl phthalate (DEHP), a plastic "softening" chemical often used in footwear, vinyl flooring, and various medical devices
- Polyvinyl chloride (PVC), a chemical used in food packaging, plastic wrap, and shower curtains
- Polyethylene terephthalate (PET), a plastics chemical added to water bottles, carpet fiber, and even chewing gum
- Urea-formaldehyde, a chemical used in particle board and plywood
- Polyurethane foam, used in pillows, cushions and mattresses

8) CHEMTRAILS

Not to be confused with normal contrails, chemtrails are those billowing releases from airplanes that don't dissipate, but rather expand and create blankets of white haze in the sky. This geoengineering pollution has been tested in some areas and found to contain high levels of aluminum, barium, and other health-damaging chemicals that, unfortunately, are difficult to avoid.

In 2004, a team of researchers from the Wyoming Institute of Technology tried to get to the bottom of the chemtrail phenomenon, examining rain and groundwater samples from Redding and other locales throughout Shasta County in Northern California. What they uncovered was a formidable laundry list of cancer-causing chemicals.

> The samples underwent numerous tests and were found to contain barium, fiberglass, radioactive thorium, mold spores, cadmium and desiccated blood. . . . Many of these substances are known to cause cancer, and cancer rates are undeniably on the rise in Shasta County. Between 1998 and 2014, the cancer rate has nearly tripled and the citizens have noticed an obvious connection.[22]

9) PROCESSED MEAT

When it comes to food, they say fresh is best. And we know that the fewer chemicals the better. But what about meat, and particularly *cured* meat that contains chemical preservatives? The World Health Organization says that eating just two ounces of processed meat per day—this includes things like hot dogs, beef jerky, sausage, and salami—increases one's risk of colorectal cancer by about 18 percent. A WHO panel of 22 scientists looked at data from more than 800 studies linking processed meat consumption cancer. Stomach, pancreatic, and colorectal cancers were all prevalent among processed-meat eaters, and the causes include exposure to carcinogenic polycyclic aromatic hydrocarbons (PAHs) as well as nitrite preservatives.

Nitrites trigger the formation of N-nitroso compounds that in animal studies have been linked to causing cancer. Cooking meats at high temperatures also results in the catalyzing of heterocyclic amines, or HCAs, which contain cancer-causing PAHs.[23]

Clean food is such an important part of living an anticancer lifestyle that many alternative cancer treatment protocols hold it in the same high esteem as the potent therapeutics they prescribe. Thomas Edison put it rightly when he said, "The doctor of the future will no longer treat the human frame with drugs, but rather will cure and prevent disease with nutrition."

CHAPTER 7

DETECTION "DOS" AND "DON'TS"

I remember thinking as I mournfully watched my parents waste away from conventional cancer treatments during the final days of their lives that I never wanted to see that happen to another family member or friend *ever* again. I didn't fully understand the ghastly repercussions of chemotherapy and radiation, and the utterly destructive effects that these treatments have on the human body. But I knew that it didn't make logical sense to "treat" any disease with known carcinogens and chemical poison, nor did it make sense to diagnose/detect cancer with methods that might actually perpetuate the disease.

Early detection isn't always beneficial, especially when the methods being used aren't always accurate—and in some cases, are even carcinogenic! Mammography is a perfect example of this: the National Cancer Institute estimates that among women under age 35, routine mammograms likely cause 75 new cases of breast cancer for every 15 they accurately identify.[1]

I'll dive further into the pitfalls of mammography later on in this chapter, but before I do I want to make it clear that early detection screenings of all kinds—at least those recommended by the cancer industry—are generally risky. Truth be told, cancer screenings are often inaccurate and many are actually *harmful*, two inconvenient truths that you'll likely never hear about from the corporate media. Rarely, if ever, do we hear about the very real risks associated with mammograms for breast cancer, PSA (prostate-specific antigen) tests for prostate cancer, colonoscopies for colon cancer, and the many other cancer screening methods commonly recommended for best-chance survival. Knowing that there was so much we weren't being told about the true nature of early detection, I continued my journey in search of answers and came to a shocking realization:

The cancer screening process is often used as a manipulation tool to herd more people into the cancer treatment fold.

What I mean is this: whether it generates false positives or causes the very cancers it's supposed to detect, early detection is typically just a ploy to sign more people up for chemotherapy and radiation. And as you now know, these treatments can spell a death sentence for those who don't truly understand what they do and how they obliterate the immune system.

CANCER IS ITS OWN CURE

Cancer is arguably one of the most misunderstood diseases on the planet. The public has largely been led to believe that if and when cancer shows up, it's necessary to unleash the chemicals and radiation to get rid of it—and fast! There's also the pervasive notion that more and frequent cancer screenings mean better chances of preventing and overcoming cancer, when in truth screenings can make the problem worse by interfering with the body's natural process of dealing with cancer cells.

I touched on this earlier, but nearly everything we've been told about cancer is flat-out wrong, as cancer is *completely normal*. Your body is fully equipped to deal with cancer all on its own, as it possesses an amazing ability to destroy the tens of thousands of new cancer cells that develop *daily*. The human immune system, when functioning optimally, is a truly remarkable wonder of creation, and not enough credit is given where credit is due.

Cancer, for all intents and purposes, is actually the ultimate remedy for extreme toxicity. It's a lot like localized inflammation when you get an infection, or a fever when you develop the flu; it's the means by which your body tries to normalize the damage caused by metabolic failure, chemical exposure, and other factors that lead to cancer.

My good friend Dr. Leonard Coldwell, a naturopathic doctor, radio host, and best-selling author who's also a medical doctor, explained it to me like this: "Cancer is the cure. People don't understand that. Cancer is there to save your life. When your body is so toxic that you are going to die of the poison, the body builds a bag and stuffs all the poison in there and locks it up—the tumor."

It might be a tough pill to swallow based on everything you thought you knew, but it's the truth. Cancer is the body's normal reaction to extreme pathogenic and toxic invasion, and cancer screenings, for all the good their proponents claim them to be, can impede this immune mechanism and actually cause cancer to spiral out of control into an eventual death sentence.

Problems arise, however, when cancer cells stop doing their job and go rogue—and perhaps calling them cancer cells in the first place is a bit of a misnomer in this regard. While it's true that our bodies always have some level of cancer cells present, the "good" kind are those that know when they're damaged and decide to either repair themselves or commit cell suicide. This is what we would call the normal cell cycle.

The "bad" kinds of cancer cells are those that continue to replicate despite being malignant, forming tumors by sapping from the body energy and nutrients that are intended for healthy cells. These are the types of cancer cells that screenings aim to detect and that treatments aim to destroy—and these are the types that are *never* okay to just leave alone, as the immune system rapidly loses its ability to naturally deal with them; outside intervention is required.

DANGERS OF MAMMOGRAMS

The modus operandi of breast cancer prevention is routine mammograms, which the American Cancer Society recommends all women over age 45 receive on an annual basis. The idea is to catch breast cancer early so it can be treated early, thus minimizing the risk of metastasis and eventual death.

But the mechanistic action of a mammogram—squeezing breast tissue between two solid plates—defies all logic if you truly understand how cancer works. If a cancer tumor really is like a bag of poison that the body has sequestered in order to neutralize and annihilate, squeezing that bag simply to detect its presence is about the worst thing you can do in terms of prevention.

"If you already have a cancer, in addition to being painful, the crushing compression the breast undergoes during a mammogram can cause the cancer to spread," says Dr. Russell Blaylock of *The Blaylock Wellness Report*.[2] "Doctors are taught that once a lump is found, you don't press it—not even during an examination—because you will cause the cancer cells to spread."

For my docuseries, I also got a chance to speak with Dr. Raymond Hilu, M.D., founder and medical director of the Hilu Institute in Spain, and he had similar thoughts on the dangers of mammograms. Compressing potentially cancerous breast tissue risks unleashing a torrent of cancer cells into outlying tissue and possibly even the bloodstream. And by the time a tumor is even detected, he told me, it's already too late to do anything about it anyway. "We hear about early detection being your best protection with mammograms. (But) by the time you see it on a mammogram, it's too late, typically. You want to catch it early and that's what this allows you to do," he explained to me, advocating instead for high-resolution blood analysis, or HRB, a safe, nontoxic diagnostic tool that amplifies the blood up to 18,000 times in order to detect free radical damage, immune dysfunction, heavy metal detoxification, and more.

Mammograms also emit ionizing radiation, which, in addition to the mechanical pressure involved with the procedure, mutates the cells it's potentially unleashing from the tumor. The Radiological Society of North America confirms that annual mammograms are directly responsible for causing breast cancer in some women.

One such type of breast cancer, ductal carcinoma in situ, or DCIS, has increased in prevalence by some 328 percent since mammography was first introduced. Statistical analyses reveal that up to 200 percent of this increase is due to a combination of the radiation and mechanical pressure involved in the mammogram procedure.

If you can believe it, the amount of radiation emitted during a single mammogram is up to 1,000 times greater than that of a typical chest X-ray. This would help explain why some cancer organizations are starting to pare down their recommendations for mammograms, especially as rates of breast cancer continue to skyrocket.[3]

And then there are the false positives, which account for more than 93 percent of all mammogram referrals, according to a paper published in *The Lancet*. Mammograms are incapable of distinguishing between healthy and malignant tissue because they simply can't provide clear and specific enough readings for doctors to make that judgment. So many women end up going through even more painful and dangerous procedures like tissue biopsies as a result of these false positives, generating more fear, anxiety, and needless treatments with chemotherapy and radiation. It's a vicious cycle that creates many more victims than it does heroes, unless you're the cancer industry itself that gets to rake in all the profits.

"Early detection is like a colonoscopy—firstly, it doesn't even get high enough to find anything important. Secondly, it pokes holes in the colon. Thirdly, those administering the treatment are unable to clean all their so-called sterile instruments in a way that won't present harm to you," says Dr. Coldwell analogously. "It's all about making money. It's not about curing you. It's not about helping you. There is not one medical doctor in the universe who can cure you."

PSA TESTS ARE LIKE MAMMOGRAMS FOR MEN

More recently, the cancer industry has been pushing the PSA test for men as a way to scope out prostate cancer. But just like mammography, this screening procedure is doing more harm than good, leaving in its wake a stream of false positives and ultimately false *hope*. The PSA test, in all truth, is mostly *worthless* because its approach to dealing with cancer completely misses the mark. Many experts say this popular blood test "poses more risks than benefits," according to *Consumer Reports.* The U.S. Preventive Services Task Force, for example, stands in bold opposition to the official cancer industry position on PSA testing, recommending doctors stop screening of all men because many more men "will experience the harms of screening and treatment of screen-detected disease than will experience the benefit."[4]

High levels of PSA can mean many other things besides cancer, yet nearly every man who scores high on the test is urged to undergo a prostate biopsy, an extremely invasive procedure that, again, like mammograms for women, can lead to the spread of cancer cells from the site of a possible tumor to the rest of the body.

As it turns out, most men have naturally occurring cancer cells in their prostates, as do women in their breasts. The immune system is fully capable of dealing with these cells on its own. Agitating them with radiation, pressure, and biopsies is like shaking an active beehive; it's definitely not something that has positive consequences.

Mammograms, biopsies, CT (computed tomography) scans: these and many other conventional screening and testing procedures for cancer are fatally flawed in the ways they attempt to deal with cancer. They're a detriment to those who undergo them, but these procedures serve the interests of the cancer industry by providing an endless stream of new patients—or more accurately, *customers*—to enrich the financial coffers of the industry players.

THE PUSH FOR SCREENING

As a brief aside, looking at how we got here, I think it's important for you to understand how cancer "awareness" is directly tied to this new-found push for everyone to be screened for cancer. It can all be traced back to the chemical industry, which invented campaigns like Breast Cancer Awareness Month (NBCAM) as a tool to compel people into getting screened, and ultimately into getting *treated*, for cancer.

Drug giant AstraZeneca, formerly a division of Imperial Chemical Industries (ICI) and manufacturer of the world's most popular breast cancer drug, tamoxifen, is the original founder of NBCAM. In partnership with the American Cancer Society, AstraZeneca came up with the idea in 1985 as a way to promote mammography as "the most effective weapon in the fight against breast cancer," to quote Wikipedia.

According to my good friend Sayer Ji over at GreenMed*Info,* the screening movement is both deceiving the general public and distracting from *actual* cancer prevention, which has nothing to do with getting mammograms. "When it comes to the breast cancer industry's emphasis on equating 'prevention' with 'early detection' through X-ray mammography, nowhere is the inherently pathological ideology of allopathic medicine more clearly evident. . . . Not only is the very ionizing radiation used to discern pathological lesions in breast tissue one of the very risk factors for the development of breast cancer, but the identification of the word 'prevention' with 'early detection' is a disingenuous way of saying that all we can do to prevent breast cancer is to detect its inevitable presence sooner than would be possible without this technology."[5]

ALTERNATIVES TO CONVENTIONAL CANCER SCREENINGS

There's certainly a time and a place for cancer screenings *when they're done right*. But the last thing your body needs is a blast of cancer-causing radiation to supposedly detect cancer, or routine scans for biomarkers of cancer that are also biomarkers of *not* cancer. There has to be a better way than what the system is currently offering, you're probably thinking by now, and the good news is: *there is*!

The following protocols aren't officially endorsed by the cancer industry, but they're far safer and much more accurate than mammography and PSA tests. Many of these I discovered for the first time during my travels over the past several years, and I'm excited to share this information with you in the hope that you and your loved ones will avoid making a screening mistake that, in a worst-case scenario, could cost you your *life*. These are the diagnostic "dos" that I would recommend any day over the conventional "don'ts:"

1) THERMOGRAPHY
Misinformation abounds as to the true nature of breast cancer and what causes it. With so much public focus on breast cancer awareness, very little attention is given to breast *health*, which we know is governed by things like clean eating, routine detoxification, energy balance, and stress reduction, among other things. These other things include *not*

blasting radiation at the breasts in the form of mammograms, which only exacerbate breast cancer risk.

Dr. Martin Bales, L.Ac., D.A.O.M., a licensed acupuncturist and certified thermologist at the Center for New Medicine in Irvine, California, has for years been administering one of the best-known alternatives to mammograms: thermograms. As its name suggests, thermography utilizes the power of infrared heat—hence the root word "therm"—to detect physiological abnormalities indicative of a possible breast cancer diagnosis. Dr. Bales's father first pioneered the technology in the late 1970s with the development of the world's first all-digital infrared camera, which was used for missile detection purposes during wartime. Its capacity to track the heat signature of missiles was applied to the field of medicine in the 1980s, which eventually gave way to thermographic medical devices.

Dr. Bales opined during a recent interview: "In the early eighties, a group of doctors approached my father and said, 'You know, we've heard the body—obviously with its (blood) circulation—we can diagnose a lot of diseases by seeing where there's hot spots and where there's cold.' He said, 'Okay, I'll make a medical version for you.'"

And the rest is history: thermography machines that identify hot spots in the breasts later hit the market, and select doctors and clinics offer it as a safe, side effect–free alternative to mammograms. "The most promising aspect of thermography is its ability to spot anomalies years before mammography," says women's health expert Christiane Northrup, M.D., about the merits of thermography. "With thermography as your regular screening tool, it's likely that you would have the opportunity to make adjustments to your diet, beliefs, and lifestyle to transform your cells before they became cancerous. Talk about true prevention."[6]

2) AMAS (ANTI-MALIGNIN ANTIBODY IN SERUM)

Earlier when I talked about the pitfalls of mammography and PSA tests in terms of their tendency to produce a high number of false positives, I was anxious to immediately bring up AMAS testing (but instead decided to save the best for last). Anti-malignin antibody in serum testing is a highly effective screening method that's capable of detecting *any* type of cancer with 95 percent accuracy after one test, and over 99 percent accuracy after two tests.

AMAS is an antibody that occurs naturally in blood serum, and it becomes elevated when any type of cancer starts to flourish and spread. It shows up first before any other anticancer antibody, which means it's technically the *earliest* cancer detection tool available. AMAS testing is nontoxic, exceptionally accurate, and can be used both for detection and monitoring.

"All cancers make anti-malignin antibody," writes Dr. Tim Smith, M.D., in his book *The GcMAF Book (2.0)*. "When our immune system identifies the presence of malignin, it starts making anti-malignin antibodies. . . . When a treatment shrinks a cancer, the AMAS will go down. . . . Normally, a healthy immune system (one with *activated* macrophages) is destroying these cancer cells as they are formed. An AMAS level that rises beyond the baseline of 135, however, tells us that the immune system is not getting rid of those new cancer cells in a timely way, and their numbers are therefore increasing. Cancer is afoot."[7]

Multicenter, double-blind clinical studies conducted by Oncolab, which offers free AMAS testing kits, show that AMAS testing is a highly effective method of both detecting cancers early and tracking their progression as a patient undergoes treatment and/or makes dietary and lifestyle changes to help bring AMAS levels back down to the normal range.[8]

3) HUMAN CHORIONIC GONADOTROPIN (HCG) URINE IMMUNOASSAY

Similar to how a pregnancy test works, an hCG urine immunoassay identifies the presence of human chorionic gonadotropin, or hCG, in the urine, which the late oncologist Dr. Manuel D. Navarro of the Navarro Medical Clinic in the Philippines discovered back in the 1950s is a biomarker of cancer. This hormone is normally released by human embryos upon conception, but it is also released by cancer cells as a cloak to get past the immune system. The higher the levels of hCG in one's urine, in other words, the greater the malignancy of a present or impending cancer.

The idea of testing for hCG was first hatched after researchers came up with the theory that cancer is associated with misplaced tropho-blastic cells, which are what compose the outer layer of the blastocysts that provide food for a developing human embryo. When these cells go awry, they begin releasing hCG that can easily be identified in blood serum and urine, the latter being what the Navarro Medical Clinic evaluates due to its superior accuracy.

Tests conducted in the 1980s found that an hCG urine immuno-assay has a remarkable success rate of about 98 percent. It can detect brain cancer as early as 29 months before the first symptoms appear; fibrosarcoma of the abdomen 27 months early; skin cancer 24 months early; and bone cancer 12 months early. "Thousands of cancer survivors have used this test over the years to keep track of their treatment(s) success and check the status of their remission," the Clinic reports. "Patients follow a simple direction for preparing a dry extract from the urine sample. The powdery extract is mailed to the Navarro Medical Clinic where the hCG testing is performed."[9]

4) ONCOBLOT TEST

You're probably starting to see a pattern emerge: cancer cells have certain unique identifying attributes that differentiate them from normal cells, and forward thinkers are figuring out what these are, how to identify them, and how to use this knowledge to help people avoid and/or overcome cancer. The ONCOblot test fits this M.O. perfectly, but rather than look for hormones in urine or antibodies in blood, it looks for a protein that only exists on the outer surfaces of certain types of cancer cells.

Dr. James Morré, a researcher from Purdue University in Indiana, first came up with the idea during his teenage years at the University of Missouri. His first job had him spraying crops with an Agent Orange derivative known as 2,4-D that eradicated out-of-control weeds in a matter of days without killing the crops they were invading, which got him thinking: What if the same concept could be applied to cancer?

This herbicide is selectively toxic, meaning it only kills target weeds, and it does so by basically giving weeds "cancer"—the cells inside these weeds are triggered to divide and multiply uncontrollably, which eventually kills them. Dr. Morré came to realize that human cancer cells have their own markers that can be selectively targeted, or at the very least selectively *identified*, and one type of marker is NOX proteins, which he's credited for being the first to discover. Dr. Morré later honed this down to a single NOX protein that he dubbed tNOX, now known as ENOX2, which only exists on the outer surfaces of malignant cancer cells. And the best part about this discovery is that each type of cancer has its own distinct form of ENOX2, which makes it quite simple to pinpoint the specific type of cancer from which a person is suffering. "The protein has a different molecular weight depending on where the cancer originated," explains Michele Cagan from the Health Sciences Institute.[10] "So the test that Morré developed not only shows whether you have cancer, it can tell you exactly where it started."

One of the weaknesses of the AMAS test that I mentioned earlier is that it can't identify precisely *where* a cancer might be forming; it can only pick up that a cancer is forming *somewhere*, which is helpful to an extent. The ONCOblot test, on the other hand, is capable of revealing a cancer's organ(s) of origin with about 96 percent accuracy.

An analysis of over 800 ONCOblots covering 26 different types of clinically confirmed cancers showed a 99.3 percent accuracy rate in detection with *no* false positives and less than 1 percent false negatives. At a cost of just $850 from the Cancer Center for Healing in Irvine, California (price subject to change), the ONCOblot test is one of the simplest and most accurate diagnostic tests for cancer available to the public.

"The ONCOblot Test has been shown to detect cancer as early as stage 0," says the Center.[11] "The limit of detection is an estimated 2 million cells (2 mm or less tumor mass, roughly the size of a pinhead) compared to several billion cells for a positive mammogram. . . . Each type of ENOX2 has a specific location (molecular weight and isoelectric point) on the blot to demonstrate ENOX2 presence and to identify the tissue of origin."

5) THYMIDINE KINASE TEST

So far, we've addressed early detection protocols that identify antibodies (AMAS), hormones (hCG), and proteins (ENOX2) in conjunction with cancer, but what about enzymes? This is what a thymidine kinase test looks for: thymidine kinase 1, or TK1, is an enzyme that repairs damaged DNA inside the body, and a 2013 study published in the journal *Cancer and Clinical Oncology* explains that it's typically associated with the proliferation of malignant cancer cells.[12]

Like the other screening methods I've already highlighted, the thymidine kinase test can be used not only to detect cancer but also to track its progression, furnishing patients and their doctors with insight into the effectiveness of a particular cancer treatment. The original version of the test looked only for TK1 in blood serum, but newer technologies can also detect it in tumor tissue. "Thymidine kinase is a cell cycle-dependent marker that can be detected in the serum of patients diagnosed with many different types of cancer," explains a review published in the journal *Expert Review of Molecular Diagnostics*.[13] These include cancers of the breast, lung, colon, skin, gastrointestinal tract, and blood.

TK1 tests are currently available to canines and other domesticated animals suspected of having cancer, but aren't generally used in humans. A number of studies have concluded that this needs to change, however, showing evidence of success across the mammalian spectrum.

A more recent study published in the journal *Anticancer Research* in 2014 suggests that TK1 testing be used in the detection and management of lung cancer. This study refers to TK1 as "a well-established cancer biomarker which is elevated in patient serum and tumor tissue of many hematological and solid tumor types,"[14] while the *Cancer and Clinical Oncology* paper dubs TK1 "a valuable cancer marker in a wide variety of solid tumors and may be considered a universal cancer marker."

The *Expert Review of Molecular Diagnostics* paper is the most frank: "Thymidine kinase assay kits should be available at low cost and could serve as an effective low cost test for the detection and progression of many types of human cancer."

6) NAGALASE TEST

While it's a fact that our immune systems are fully equipped to make mincemeat out of cancer, certain conditions must be met in order for this to happen. The macrophages that scope out, attack, and eradicate cancer cells must first be activated by GcMAF, short for group specific component macrophage activating factor, in order for this immune response to occur and be effective. One of the reasons why this often isn't the case is because cancer cells have learned how to outsmart the immune system, producing a substance known as Nagalase that blocks the production of GcMAF and effectively turns macrophages into macro*failures*. In his book *The GcMAF Book 2.0*, Dr. Smith describes macrophages that lack GcMAF as being "zombies" stuck in a state of suspended animation.

Nagalase is basically an enzyme secreted by cancer cells as they go about their business of forming into a tumor. It attacks the extracellular matrix of GcMAF, rendering it impotent and incapable of generating an appropriate immune response to the invading cancer. "GcMAF is the protein that activates macrophages and jump-starts the entire immune response," Dr. Smith writes. "To sabotage the immune system and put the macrophages to sleep, all cancers and viruses make Nagalase, the enzyme that blocks production of GcMAF. In the absence of GcMAF, cancers, HIV, and other viruses can grow unimpeded."[15]

The interesting thing about Nagalase is that both cancer cells *and viruses* produce it, which to some is a downside to Nagalase testing specifically for cancer. But there's an easy way around this: viruses subside after a time, bringing Nagalase levels back down to baseline, whereas cancers continue to produce it at an increasingly exponential rate over time. A series of Nagalase tests conducted over several weeks or months will provide clarity as to whether or not a patient is dealing with a virus or cancer. And because Nagalase shows up early, long before cancer cells are able to metastasize, it's an invaluable tool for catching cancers early and eradicating them. "If all new cancers were detected early by regular Nagalase testing, we could reverse them with GcMAF—long before X-rays could find them—and put cancer out of business once and for all," Dr. Smith adds.

The solution to Nagalase, which I'll expand upon more in later chapters, is to reintroduce GcMAF into the body via a series of simple injections. There's also newer research suggesting that special

GcMAF-producing cultures in yogurt may provide similar benefits without the needle.[16]

7) HIGH-RESOLUTION BLOOD (HRB) ANALYSIS

Leviticus 17:11 states that the life of the body is in the blood, and from a scientific perspective, we can now say with certainty precisely why: our blood is what keeps our bodies alive, transporting oxygen, nutrients, and immune factors to cells while pulling carbon dioxide from cell tissue.

When something goes wrong inside the body, chances are it began in the blood. And thanks to modern technology, we now have the ability to examine blood closely to measure vitamin and mineral levels, protein content, and chemical composition in order to diagnose disease.

An advanced blood analysis can also come in handy for early detection of cancer, which is what Dr. Raymond Hilu of the Hilu Institute in Malaga, Spain, has been doing since 2008. He explained to me during an interview for my docuseries how his method of high-resolution blood analysis, or HRB, accurately maps the structure of blood in order to identify certain abnormalities indicative of cancer. "This is a high-resolution cellular study of the blood," he told me. "You just need a couple of drops from the finger. . . . We magnify the sample up to sixty-five thousand times, so I'm able to see what's happening even inside the cells. It gives me a very good idea of the imbalances, deficiencies, irregular morphologies, and the contents of the blood serum. So whatever is wrong, I take note of it, and try to put it right. It's as simple as that."

Though not originally developed as a cancer diagnostic tool per se, HRB analysis provides an exceptionally accurate look into the complex workings of the cellular system, allowing practitioners trained in what to look for the unique opportunity to extrapolate this data into a preliminary diagnosis. The method is highly effective at detecting the presence of cancer cells long before they have the opportunity to develop into full-blown tumors. Dr. Hilu refers to these cellular imbalances as being "precancerous," treatable early on before a cancer metastasizes.

"That's the beginning of any disease," he says, noting that HRB analysis can detect some cancers up to five years in advance. "Things start to go wrong on a cellular level—and this is where the microscope becomes a very useful tool. Because we start seeing these irregularities before the disease appears, even cancer, years in advance. So we can prevent diseases from happening."

Even if a patient is already suffering from a more advanced form of cancer, he says, HRB analysis can pick up on the particular cellular imbalances that caused it, making a customized treatment plan that much easier to develop. And according to Dr. Hilu, preventing *and treating* cancer is what HRB Analysis is all about: "Of course, if the patient is already suffering from cancer, we will see the imbalances that the patient is suffering and the things that are making cancer grow worse and we try to correct them as well. So it's useful to treat, but mainly I love to use this tool to prevent the disease from happening." [17]

These are just a few examples of the types of tools that emerging science is unveiling as adjuncts to—or better yet, *replacements for*— the more traditional radiation screenings with which you're probably familiar. Each of the diagnostic methods I've covered for you here is safe, highly effective, and exceptionally accurate.

There's a peace of mind that comes with knowing that you aren't poisoning your body in the process of trying to heal it. That's why these screening tools exist, and I hope you'll share this information with your loved ones to help them avoid falling victim to the radiation- and surgery-based screening methods that harm more than they help.

CHAPTER 8

HOW CAN I PREVENT CANCER?

It might sound a tad cliché, but it's true that the best way to treat cancer is to avoid getting it in the first place. And when I say cancer, based on what we've covered thus far, I'm talking about the prolific, metastasizing kind that's already exceeded what the immune system is capable of handling on its own, demanding some serious outside intervention.

This is the kind of cancer you *don't* want to develop, and the key to keeping it in check, or what we would call active cancer prevention, is to adopt a holistic, anticancer *lifestyle* that supports the health of the three primary components that make up a human being: mind, body, and spirit. You probably thought I was only going to focus on food and exercise here, but truth be told your thoughts and the things you believe are just as important as what you eat and how active you are in terms of cancer prevention. My primary focus will indeed be centered around diet, exercise, and supplementation as a primary means to prevent cancer. But I'd also like to delve a bit into the emotional and spiritual aspects of holistic health because both of these are vitally interconnected to the physical state of being.

Nutrition is by and large the most critical aspect of cancer prevention because food is the literal "fuel" that our bodies use to repair and maintain cells, build immunity, produce energy, and fend off disease. When you aren't eating enough of the right foods, or when you're scarfing down too many of the *wrong* ones, your body becomes increasingly more prone to suffering a functional breakdown; this just makes common sense.

The vast complexity of the human body, however, is demarcated by the simple fact that it operates as a single organism *with many unique parts*. The head isn't greater than the hand, just as the heart isn't greater than the liver. Each system of the body is vitally important in its own right for the complete organism to function properly as it should, and nutrition is quite obviously what bridges the gap between these individual parts and the systemic whole.

But your emotional and spiritual health also help undergird this bridge. Dr. Rosy Daniel, M.D., an integrative medicine specialist who founded and currently serves as medical director of the famed Bristol Cancer Help Centre in the United Kingdom, is a firm believer in what I like to call the holistic cancer prevention approach, which takes into account all three aspects of human existence: the physical, the mental, and the spiritual.

Dr. Daniel developed a unique health coaching approach called "Health Creation" that addresses what she says is the true cause of practically all chronic illnesses, including heart disease, obesity, and cancer: destructive lifestyle choices—or in her own words, miscreant "health-defining behavior."[1] Health-defining behavior, of course, involves a whole lot more than just one's eating habits; it also encompasses thought patterns and spiritual growth, two major focuses of her practice. "When people grow dispirited or crushed, or have lost their way in life, medicine becomes much less effective," she writes in her book *The Cancer Prevention Book*, highlighting the ever-evolving and expanding field of psychoneuroimmunology, or PNI, which looks at the inextricable link between mind and body.[2] "Conversely, when they become excited or motivated, living purposeful lives over which they feel they have control, the incidence of serious disease falls and the success of treatment greatly increases."

In other words, your dietary choices only go as far in protecting your body against disease as your thought processes and spiritual condition allow them to, and vice versa: the foods you eat and the level of physical activity in which you engage will either help or hinder your mental and spiritual progress because food and exercise directly affect brain function, which is also a key component to spiritual understanding.

SPIRITUAL, EMOTIONAL GROUNDING FOR CANCER PREVENTION

Case in point: the health and well-being of me and my family is just as much a function of our diet as it is of our Christian faith. The spiritual anchor to which we're moored is what keeps us grounded during the storms of life, providing a peace that passes all understanding. And this peace is what helps us keep our stress levels in check, which in turn helps minimize the excess bodily release of adrenaline and cortisol, both of which can damage the immune system in too high amounts.

For us, knowing that our earthly afflictions are momentary and light and that they serve a greater purpose beyond just the temporal creates a unique sense of spiritual *stability* in our lives. And this stability spills over into the emotional and physical realms by helping eliminate anxiety, worry, and stress; each of these mental states, in case you weren't aware, release inflammatory stress hormones that can damage the body and lead to chronic disease.

This isn't to say that all physical discomfort can be avoided like magic simply by tapping into the spiritual realm. To the contrary, a genuinely healthy spiritual state grounded in truth acts as an emotional stabilizer, which in turn lends itself to an improved physical state that would otherwise be overshadowed and burdened by insecurities, worry, stress, and other physically taxing states of being.

A 1993 study published in the journal *Health Progress* puts it like this: "Spiritual health is that aspect of our well-being which organizes the values, the relationships, and the meaning and purpose of our lives. Patients and healthcare professionals alike have experienced a growing recognition of the importance of spiritual health as a foundation for physical health and well-being."[3]

Emotional wounds are likewise taxing to the physical body, which is why many integrative and holistic practitioners work closely with patients to help them overcome and move past these damaging strongholds. The Breast Cancer Conqueror protocol likens the etymological nature of the word *emotion* to "energy in motion," and I think there's definitely some truth to this.[4] When you're stuck in an unhealthy emotional state, the protocol warns, the energy systems of your physical body become damaged or impeded.

When we're anxious or stressed, our bodies accumulate tension. We quickly move from a relaxed state to a wound-up, apprehensive one, and the physical damage this causes when left unchecked is both tangible and substantial. Have you ever heard the phrase "bottling up your emotions"? There are very real consequences to holding on to unhealthy emotions for too long a period of time: they become bottled up, resulting in physical manifestations of illness. Breast Cancer Conqueror puts it like this: "Have you ever felt stressed out about something and you noticed that your neck muscles or jaw felt really tight? Remember feeling that pit in your stomach or that ache in your solar plexus? That is an example of your 'e-motions' or 'energy in motion' getting stuck. . . . We now have proof that your DNA contracts and relaxes in response to your mood."

If you've never heard of this type of thing before, you're not alone; I, too, had an eye-opening experience the first time I made the connection between what's going on both upstairs and in my soul to what I was feeling and experiencing physically. As I gained a greater understanding of *how* these aspects of my being are interconnected, *why* I was feeling the way I did made more sense.

PHYSICAL EXERCISE FOR CELL OXYGENATION AND DETOXIFICATION

It's one of those "which came first: the chicken or the egg?" conundrums. Is a bad spiritual and/or mental state responsible for causing physical ailments, or do preexisting physical ailments end up leading to a bad spiritual and/or mental state? And what about physical *exercise*: Is a sedentary lifestyle the *cause* or the *result* of a poor emotional and/or spiritual state of being?

In many ways, I believe that *all* of these scenarios have some truth to them, and here are some reasons why, as well as some additional tips for breaking this toxic and destructive cycle:

1) SWEATING DETOXIFIES THE BODY OF MIND-ALTERING CHEMICALS

One of the main reasons why regular exercise is such a crucial weapon in the cancer prevention arsenal is that exercise causes your body to sweat, which is one of the primary means by which our bodies eliminate toxins. In addition to their potential carcinogenicity, these toxins directly interfere with brain neurochemistry, altering how we think and perceive the world around us.

Conditions like "brain fog" and relapsed memory, which may also include more serious mental problems like dementia, are increasingly being linked to persistent internal toxicity, as chemical poisons remain inside the body rather than get "flushed" out through sweat as they're supposed to, eventually leading to disease.

The body has two different types of sweat glands: eccrine, which are found all over your body; and apocrine, which are found only on the scalp, armpits, and genital area. The roughly 3 million sweat glands found on your body help regulate your autonomic nervous system, raise body temperature, and perhaps most importantly, expel toxins.

Sweating also releases antimicrobial substances like dermicidin that keep your skin flora in check and help prevent skin infections. That's right: sweat is actually a key component of your body's immune system, which is why you need to get it going regularly to help keep your body clean and disease free. "Sweating has long been perceived to promote health," explains one study published in the *Journal of Environmental and Public Health*, "not only accompanying exercise but also with heat. Worldwide traditions and customs include Roman baths, Aboriginal sweat lodges, Scandinavian saunas (dry heat; relative humidity from 40% to 60%), and Turkish baths (with steam)."

Concerning the elimination of toxins like arsenic, cadmium, mercury, and lead, the same study adds, "Sweating is not only observed to enhance excretion of the toxic elements of interest in this paper, but also may increase excretion of diverse toxicants . . . or in particular persistent flame retardants and bisphenol-A."[5]

2) AEROBIC EXERCISE GETS BLOOD FLOWING AND OXYGEN MOVING

As a former bodybuilder, I'm quite familiar with the cardiovascular benefits of both strength and aerobic training. When you exert your body through rigorous exercise, your raise your heart rate and maximize your oxygen uptake, which benefits your heart, lungs, and blood vessels. Whether you like to bike, walk, run, swim, play sports, or even dance, engaging in continuous physical activity for at least 20 minutes daily, three times a week, at 60 percent or more of your maximum heart rate will help you feel better, sleep better, think better, and experience a much higher quality of life.

The general consensus is that we need to engage in at least 150 minutes per week of moderate aerobic activity—which includes things like brisk walking, swimming, and mowing the lawn—or 75 minutes per week of vigorous aerobic activity: think soccer, basketball, running, and Zumba.[6]

Whatever you can do to get your heart pumping at the target rate for your age—a 20-year-old would want to attain a heart rate of between 130 and 150 beats per minute (bpm), while a 60-year-old would aim for between 104 and 120 bpm[7]—is ideal for the purposes of disease prevention.

Remember, in order to get oxygen delivered to all the right places in your body, you absolutely *must* exert yourself and get that heart rate going on a regular basis. Oxygen is a requirement for cell nourishment, energy production, waste breakdown and elimination, detoxification, nutrient metabolism, pH balance, and immune protection, so don't neglect it in your pursuit of better health.

3) REBOUNDING FOR YOUR LYMPHS

People often ask me if there's one exercise in particular that fully encompasses both the heart rate and detoxification aspects of body movement. What I tell them is that while all aerobic exercise is beneficial, rebounding is *especially* beneficial because it activates the lymph system in such a way as to maximize the elimination of both toxins and cancer cells.

A rebounder is basically a mini-trampoline that, because of how it moves the body, is one of the most effective ways to optimize the lymphatic system. Making up about 25 percent of white blood cell content, lymphocytes, the primary cells of the lymphatic system, draw out and eliminate abnormal body cells, including those that have become cancerous.

Unlike your blood, which is constantly circulating and working to filter out toxins from your tissue and cells regardless of your level of physical activity, your lymph only functions when you're physically active. This is why the sedentary nature of most people in the modern world is literally killing them: the average person's lymph simply isn't able to do its job, which means sickness and possible early death.

As I explained in my earlier book *Cancer: Step Outside the Box*, rebounding for just 10 to 20 minutes daily can help increase lymph function thirtyfold, and the movement of lymphocytes fivefold. It's an extremely low-impact form of aerobic exercise that offers unparalleled benefits; you essentially get the biggest bang for your buck, and your time, by using a rebounder.

4) WORK THOSE MUSCLES

I'm also a huge fan of circuit weight training because one of the things I learned throughout my bodybuilding career is that, when done properly, combining aerobic workouts with resistance training is an easy and efficient way to strengthen your heart, lungs, and immune system while simultaneously building muscle and shedding fat.

Circuit training is pretty much what it sounds like: you work through a circuit of weight machines for a set period of time—typically no more than about 45 minutes total—using lighter weights to achieve a higher number of repetitions, about 20 per exercise. Each exercise should be performed slowly with focus on the "negative" aspect of the movement; i.e., the downward motion of a dumbbell curl as opposed to the upward, lifting motion. In a nutshell, circuit training is meant to be an intense yet lower-weight workout regimen that increases your heart rate and builds muscle while minimizing oxidative damage due to decreased blood and oxygen flow to your vital organs—a condition known as hypoxia.

Depending on your physical abilities, higher-weight hypoxia training may not necessarily be a detriment, according to a recent study published in *Immunology and Cell Biology*.[8] But a lower-weight routine with higher reps is what I would recommend for the average person trying to avoid cancer and other chronic diseases.

5) AVOID CANCER-CAUSING TOXINS WHENEVER POSSIBLE

Just because your body is designed to eliminate toxins doesn't mean you should just throw caution to the wind when it comes to casual exposure to them. In light of this, the food and beverages you consume are critical to your overall wellbeing.

Yet the sad reality is that much of what the average person consumes as "food" is really just a hodgepodge of processed, food-like *chemicals* that disagree with the body's natural physiology, and are thus a source of nutritional grief. There are literally *tens of thousands* of chemicals being peddled as food, and many of these have never undergone rigorous safety review, which means we know *very little* about how they affect the body. At the same time, independent researchers and laboratories have studied quite a number of the most common ones, especially those suspected of causing cancer. Many of these are probably familiar territory if you're accustomed to healthy eating, so you can think of the following list as a fresh and helpful reminder about what to *avoid* at all costs:

1. *Hydrogenated and partially hydrogenated vegetable oils.* By artificially injecting hydrogen molecules into liquid oils, chemical manufacturers are able to turn these oils solid so they'll last longer on the shelf like naturally solid fats such as palm and coconut oils, butter, and lard. But hydrogenated and partially hydrogenated oils are "trans" fats, which have been shown to raise LDL, or "bad," cholesterol levels while increasing the risk of heart disease. "The problem with trans fatty acids is that your body doesn't know what to do with them," says Dr. Brian Olshanksy, M.D., a

University of Iowa Health Care Professor of Internal Medicine.[9] "Trans fatty acids may help preserve food so that it tastes good, but your body can't break them down and use them correctly. . . . Normal fats are very supple and pliable, but the trans fatty acid is a stiff fat that can build up in the body and create havoc. The chemical recipe for a trans fatty acid involves putting hydrogen atoms in the wrong place. It's like making a plastic."

Trans fats are incapable of binding with oxygen because they destroy the vital electron cloud around cells that enables this process. As a result, they end up clogging arteries, preventing the free flow of blood and lymph, and damaging heart tissue, among other things. You'll typically find trans fats and hydrogenated oils in snack foods like cookies and chips, packaged baked goods, fried foods, muffins, and even some cereals.

2. *Refined sugars.* Around the time I published my last book, high-fructose corn syrup (HFCS) was in almost *every-thing*. It still is, to a large extent, but food manufacturers are starting to catch on to the fact that more people than ever before are now trying to avoid this highly processed, supersweet goo, which has prompted many companies to make the switch to "all-natural cane sugar."

Cane sugar is admittedly less toxic than HFCS since it doesn't inhibit the ability of the pancreas to produce insulin. But it's still a processed form of sugar that places a heavy burden on the body. Researchers at the University of California–San Francisco found that sugar contributes to roughly 35 million deaths every year worldwide: an astounding figure that far exceeds the total number of deaths resulting from heart disease, stroke, COPD, lower respiratory infections, HIV/AIDS, diarrheal disease, diabetes, hypertensive heart disease, tracheal bronchus, and lung cancer *combined*, according to World Health Organization statistics.[10]

Sugar also acts as fuel for cancer cells, feeding their anaerobic lust to *ferment*. Dr. Mark Sircus of the International Medical Veritas Association says sugar and cancer "are locked in a death grip,"[11] and science proves this. Research published in the journal *Proceedings of the National Academy of Sciences* in 2009 was the first to show that sugar "feeds" tumors, drawing from scientific data long buried from nearly 100 years ago. "It's been known since 1923 that tumor cells use a lot more glucose than normal cells," stated Don Ayer, Ph.D., an investigator at the Huntsman Cancer Institute and professor at the University of Utah's Department of Oncological Science.[12]

This is why any credible anticancer treatment protocol will advise abstaining from sugar consumption because doing so not only starves cancer cells, but also creates a metabolic chain reaction leading to cancer cell death. Sugar is also a *cause* of cancer due to its inflammatory properties.

3. *Aspartame, MSG, and "excitotoxins."* If you've ever visited a Chinese fast food joint, you may have seen a sign in the window saying "No MSG." This is to let customers know that the restaurant doesn't add a chemical known as monosodium glutamate to its food dishes, since many people have a bad reaction to this additive. MSG is a salt derivative of the amino acid glutamic acid. It makes foods taste fresher and more savory than they otherwise would, but this comes with a catch. MSG is one of the unhealthiest

substances you can put in your body, worse than alcohol, nicotine, and even many pharmaceutical drugs.

Invented in 1908, MSG mimics the natural flavor-enhancing properties of certain seaweed derivatives, but it also targets the one vulnerability in the blood-brain barrier—the hypothalamus—allowing excitotoxins to enter the brain and cause cell damage. Dr. Russell Blaylock talks all about excitotoxins in his book *Excitotoxins: The Taste That Kills*, explaining how these Trojan horse chemicals slip by the brain's protective defenses and latch on to neuron receptors, "exciting" them to such a degree that they eventually die. Many people who consume excitotoxins report things like headaches, depression, and heart problems.

MSG specifically has also been linked to obesity as it causes the pancreas to produce upwards of *three times* the normal amount of insulin. Some food manufacturers attempt to hide the presence of MSG in their products by calling it something else, including under the following names:[13]

- Glutamic acid and anything containing "glutamate"
- Anything "hydrolyzed"
- Anything "protein" or "protein" fortified, including "textured"
- Calcium and sodium caseinate
- Anything with "yeast"
- Anything with "enzymes" or "enzyme modified"
- Anything "fermented" or containing "protease"
- Gelatin
- Soy sauce and soy sauce "extract"
- Natural flavors and flavorings

And then there's the ubiquitous artificial sweetening chemical aspartame that many people throughout the world have been hoodwinked into believing is healthier and less fattening than sugar. Like MSG, aspartame is an excitotoxin that damages brain cells, but on a much more prolific scale: FDA data shows that more than 75 percent of all adverse reactions reported in conjunction with food stem from aspartame consumption.

Originally developed as a biowarfare chemical, aspartame has long been recognized as a neurotoxin. But through lobbying sleight of hand, it somehow gained FDA approval as a sweetening chemical back in the 1980s, and is now present in soft drinks, chewing gums, mints, candies, sauces, and more.[14] Composed of methanol (wood alcohol) and two types of amino acids, aspartic acid and phenylalanine, aspartame is an interesting bird. Despite containing natural amino acids as part of its composition, aspartame's methanol component is broken down by the body and turned into formaldehyde, a known carcinogen. Sold under the brand names NutraSweet, Equal, Equal Spoonful, AminoSweet, and Equal-Measure, aspartame has been scientifically linked to causing dementia, diabetes, mental retardation, multiple sclerosis, chronic fatigue syndrome, birth defects, Parkinson's disease, and fibromyalgia, as well as cancers of the brain and lymph nodes.[15]

4. *GMOs and crop pesticides.* Ever since they were first introduced in 1996, genetically modified organisms have remained controversial, not only because they aren't labeled but also because their safety profile is questionable at best. Countless animal studies have linked their consumption to gastrointestinal disorders and immune dysfunction, while

some GMO technologies like Bt (*Bacillus thuringiensis*) are said to continue reproducing in the gut indefinitely.

Here's what we know conclusively about the nature of GMOs that should give you pause:

1) In less than a decade after the first GMOs were brought to market, the number of Americans with three or more chronic illnesses more than *doubled*. These conditions include things like food allergies, autism, reproductive disorders, and digestive problems.[16]

2) Pesticide and herbicide chemicals like Roundup (glyphosate) that are sprayed on GMOs have been linked to tumor growths both inside (organ cancer) and outside (skin cancer) the body, as well as premature death.[17]

3) Practically none of the foreign genes inserted into GMOs, which include bacterial and viral components, have been tested on humans in conjunction with the foods they eat. Nobody really knows what these substances are doing to humans, let alone the cascade of collateral damage caused by mutations to DNA and genetic expression inside the plants themselves.[18]

4) The vast majority of all corn (about 92 percent), soybeans (about 94 percent), and cotton (about 94 percent) grown in the U.S. are GMO. Most canola, sugar beets, and papaya are also GMO, as are their derivatives; "sugar," for instance, when seen on a food label, is more often than not sugar derived from GMO sugar beets, unless otherwise indicated.

"There is no monitoring of GMO-related illnesses and no long-term animal studies," explains Jeffrey Smith's Institute for Responsible Technology, one of the world's leading sources of GMO science. "Heavily invested biotech corporations are gambling with the health of our nation for profit."[19]

Other sources of toxic exposure worth avoiding include:

- *Nonstick cookware* that contains chemicals like Teflon, PFOA (perfluorooctanoic acid), and other synthetic polymer plastics that are linked to elevated cholesterol levels, thyroid damage, weakened immunity, and liver inflammation.[20]

- *Microwaves*, which denature food and damage the molecular structure of nutrients, according to research conducted by Dr. Hans Hertel.[21]

- *Bleached, refined, and "enriched" flour*, which is stripped of all of its nutrients and "fortified" with synthetic ones, including folic acid, a toxic folate impostor.[22]

- *Conventional produce*, which is sprayed with carcinogenic weed killers and pesticides. The Environmental Working Group's "Dirty Dozen," a compilation of the worst produce items based on pesticide contamination, includes conventional strawberries, apples, nectarines, peaches, celery, grapes, cherries, spinach, tomatoes, sweet bell peppers, cherry tomatoes, and cucumbers.[23]

- *Toxic personal care products*. There's so much here that this could be an entire chapter in itself. But my recommendation is to take a look at EWG's Skin Deep Cosmetics Database to learn more about which specific ingredients to avoid, and which brands use better ones.[24]

- *Soy*, which Dr. William Wong, N.D., Ph.D., says is a poison. Not only are this proliferative bean and its various derivatives estrogenic, it's also a nutrient *destroyer*.[25]

- *Plastics*. Whether it's polycarbonate (PC), bisphenol-A (BPA), polyvinyl chloride (PVC or vinyl), or some other petroleum-based plastic or plastic chemical, chances are it's not good for you.

- *Nitrites*, which preserve meat but also feed cancer cells—avoid them!
- *Fluoride*, a chemical halogen added to many public water supplies that's been linked to cancer of the bone, bladder, and lungs.[26]
- *Organochlorines*, which are chemical by-products of water chlorination. Filtering your drinking water and swimming in salt water rather than chlorine-treated pools will help you avoid these.[27]

HEALTHY NUTRITION AND LIFESTYLE

Now that you have a much more solid footing in understanding what you need to *avoid*, I'd like to offer some recommendations on what to *embrace* as part of a healthy lifestyle centered around cancer prevention. Nutrition will be the primary focus here, as this is *the* most important piece of the anticancer puzzle. But I'll also briefly address the importance of rest and fluid intake.

In a general sense, proper nutrition is categorized by foods that are dense in vitamins and minerals, free of toxic contaminants, and as close to nature as possible. This means foods like organic, non-GMO produce and meats from animals raised the way nature intended: grass fed as opposed to grain fed. In a much more specific sense, it means embracing the types of anticancer foods and herbs that have been scientifically shown to help balance internal terrain and create conditions that are unfavorable to the development of cancer and other chronic diseases.

"For cancer to go forward, the cell nucleus and the genetic material has to mutate, so that's very much a nutritional issue," says Dr. Daniel, whose main focus in cancer treatment is also centered around nutrition. "It means that you don't have the right plant foods, particularly . . . so we don't get the plant factors into our bodies, and the cell therefore is at risk of mutating the genetic material."

Chris Woollams's Rainbow Diet embodies this concept, as it's basically a traditional Mediterranean diet composed primarily of rich and colorful fruits and vegetables, a variety of nuts and seeds, lots of extra virgin olive oil, and fatty fish. It also includes high amounts of other healthy fats and even moderate wine consumption, along with some meat if you're more of a carnivore. Excluded from the diet are cheap carbohydrates and refined sugar, both of which destroy health.[28]

There are certain tweaks I would make to the Rainbow Diet, of course, including its arbitrary restrictions on red meat. Meat from grass-fed, pasture-raised animals contains high levels of omega-3 fats and other nutrients that you simply don't find in high enough amounts from most plants. I'm also a fan of raw milk, particularly from goats, sheep, and if you can find it, *camels*. Raw milk is loaded with probiotic bacteria and enzymes that aid in food digestion, nutrient assimilation, and overall gut health, which is critical in cancer prevention.

You also need to make sure you're drinking plenty of clean, fluoride- and chlorine-free water every day. Research published in the *Journal of Clinical Oncology* found that cancer risk is inversely associated with fluid intake, meaning the *more* you stay hydrated, the *less* likely you are to get sick.[29]

The same is true for sleep, which is when the body undergoes the most significant aspects of self-maintenance. Proper rest is necessary for perpetuating a healthy sleep-wake cycle, also known as circadian rhythm, which is what governs hormone balance, energy production, cell and tissue repair, and waste removal. One University of Chicago study found that lack of sleep inhibits the normal production of insulin, which we know is factor in metabolic disorder and diabetes.[30] Taken to its logical end, lack of sleep can result in insulin resistance, which various other studies have identified as a factor in cancer development.

DON'T FORGET THE ENZYMES

I'll get into more specifics about herbal supplementation and diet in the next chapter. But first I'd like to cover one more essential in the cancer prevention department: enzymes. Enzymes break down the foods we eat and ready them for digestion; without enzymes, our bodies couldn't effectively absorb nutrients, and the unfortunate reality is that our modern food supply is largely depleted of enzymes.

If your nutrient requirements were a stool with three legs, one of these legs would be enzymes, and the other two would be vitamins and minerals. Vitamins and minerals require enzymes in order to provide benefits, just as enzymes require vitamins and minerals to catalyze nutrients for assimilation. Dr. Tim O'Shea of The Doctor Within puts it like this:

> In the wacky marketplace of today's food supplements, it's like we're assaulted on all sides by people screaming Vitamins!, others yelling Minerals!, and others hollering Enzymes! as though each one alone were the Magic Bullet that can cure anything. The real ideas are cooperation, synergy, co-factoring. Nothing exists in isolation in the body. . . . An enzyme without co-factors has no enzyme activity. Enzymes are known to have very specific jobs to do. Their activity is compared to keys that must fit certain locks.[31]

Enzymes occur naturally in many foods, but they're also easily destroyed by high heat, chemicals, processing, and other factors. This is why a back-to-nature approach that focuses on eating clean, chemical-free, *raw* foods is so important; non-denatured foods have the highest enzyme content, and when they're grown and prepared in harmony with the earth, they also contain the highest amounts of vitamin and minerals to synergize with these enzymes.

Enzymes give life to the foods we eat. Without them, food is literally "dead" and incapable of fortifying our bodies with nutrition, energy, strength, and immunity. Many of the healing protocols I'm about to introduce to you would be fatally crippled without enzymes—they're that important. So keep this in mind, especially as we discuss anticancer nutritional protocols.

Part III
Successful Treatment Protocols

CHAPTER 9

HERBAL REMEDIES, DETOXIFICATION, AND DIET

Hopefully what you've gathered so far is that *prevention* is the preeminent goal when it comes to dealing with cancer. And prevention, as we've now covered, involves taking an active role in caring for your mind, your soul, and your body: a three-pronged approach to health that's most effectively executed by concertedly addressing emotional and spiritual distress for peace of mind, cleaning up your diet and overcoming nutritional deficiencies, minimizing toxic exposure in all areas of your life, and balancing your hormones with proper rest and hydration.

Each of these is important for maintaining the highest quality of life possible while minimizing your risk of cancer. But what do you do if you already *have* cancer? The first and most obvious answer is to try to identify what caused it in the first place and make the appropriate lifestyle changes to avoid exacerbating it. But you also have to aggressively deal with the cancer itself so it doesn't take over your body, which is the primary focus of this last segment of the book.

All the prevention tactics I've outlined thus far still apply, of course. But depending on the type of cancer from which you're suffering, a more aggressive remediation approach may be necessary. No matter what, remember that you *do* have options besides chemotherapy and radiation, and you shouldn't be frightened into taking these treatments when there are viable alternatives that effectively get the job done while respecting your body.

The cancer treatments I'm about to introduce you to are *herbal* in nature, which means they're among the most easily accessible options available to patients who can freely buy or grow them without necessarily having to visit a clinic or consult with a doctor (though it's important to remember that any formative cancer treatment protocol, including herbs, *should* be administered with the help and under the supervision of a qualified physician for optimal results).

After we cover herbs, I'll dive right into other progressive cancer treatments that involve the use of things like sound, light, oxygen, heat, electromagnetic frequencies, essential oils, enzymes, and more that have helped people all over the world heal from cancer. While these methods aren't an absolute guarantee of a cure, the science behind them, including actual clinical results verifying that they've eradicated tumors and associated markers of cancer in a large percentage of cases, suggests that they're the *best* options available when it comes to treating cancer.

ESSIAC TEA

In 1988 my late grandmother, Helen Cade, or "Mama Helen" as we affectionately called her, was first diagnosed with terminal cancer. I'll never forget helping this God-fearing woman prepare a special herbal concoction in her kitchen that she would take several times daily as treatment for her cancer, and that helped her live for years beyond what the doctors said she would.

When Mama Helen wasn't selflessly witnessing to others about the gospel of Jesus Christ, whom she so passionately served as a labor of love, she was busy in her kitchen brewing up this Essiac tea, as it's called, having gotten the secret recipe from who knows where. I distinctly recall watching this fascinating tea mixture boil and decoct on the stove before we poured it into amber-tinted bottles for storage in the refrigerator.

Mama Helen knew the tea worked, and so did I. It was evident in her daily vibrancy, which, had she chosen chemotherapy or radiation instead, probably would have left her ill and bedridden. But she thrived for another *10 years* on Essiac tea before eventually stopping the regimen—to this day, I'm still not sure why she chose to do this—and inevitably succumbing to the final outcome of old age: death. But her faithful use of the tea over roughly a decade's time was an inspiration to me, and it's what first got me started down the path of alternative treatments for cancer. Mama Helen must have heard through the grapevine about this particular herbal remedy, which was popularized back in 1922 by a Canadian nurse, Rene Caisse, who learned about it from one of her patients.

The patient, who had previously been diagnosed with breast cancer, explained to her that an Indian medicine man had offered up the remedy as a cure for cancer. Hearing this, Nurse Caisse decided to test it on her aunt, who had been diagnosed with terminal stomach cancer and told she only had six months to live. The tea worked like a charm: Nurse Caisse's aunt lived for another 20 years. Similar success was seen with Nurse Caisse's mom, who had been diagnosed with terminal liver cancer and told she only had two months to live—she lived for another 18 years!

Word got around, and Nurse Caisse quickly became one of the most popular physicians in her area, treating up to 600 patients *per week* before eventually closing up her practice due to relentless harassment from the medical establishment. But prior to this, she was given the opportunity to treat 30 terminal cancer patients under the direction of five medical doctors at Northwestern University Medical School in Chicago, who concluded based on their observations that Essiac tea "prolonged life, shrank tumors, and relieved pain."[1]

The Essiac tea treatment became so popular that in 1938, more than 55,000 of Nurse Caisse's Canadian supporters signed a petition to have it designated as an official cancer treatment in Canada. These efforts failed, and Caisse kept the formula for her tea under lock and key for many years as protection, until finally releasing it to her close friend and confidant Dr. Charles Brusch, director of the prestigious Brusch Clinic and personal physician to former President John F. Kennedy.

Having suffered from lower bowel cancer and using Essiac to successfully treat it, Dr. Brusch stated (in an interview with Dr. Gary Glum) about the therapy: "I know Essiac has curing potential. It can lessen the condition of the individual, control it, and it can cure it."

Nurse Caisse later handed over the recipe for her tea to the Resperin Corporation of Toronto, which she tasked with testing, manufacturing, and distributing it to people in need—a charge that Resperin has honored ever since with its continued sale and distribution of Resperin's Original Caisse Formula Tea product.[2]

Nurse Caisse was never about the money; she had built a trusted reputation for literally *giving* Essiac tea away to her patients. She *never* published the recipe herself because she feared others might try to capitalize on it for greedy purposes. Only in recent years do we have access to this sacred recipe thanks to the selfless efforts of devoted historians who've carefully pieced it together in the public interest.[3]

I can tell you plainly that Essiac tea contains just four simple ingredients. But before I list them, you should know that the *preparation* instructions are just as important as the formula itself. Unlike traditional tea infusions, Essiac tea is a *decoction*, meaning it involves extracting the *essence* of the roots, bark, and seeds of plant material, which includes things like mineral salts, bitter principles, and other "hard" materials that require boiling and extensive steeping to extract.

A decoction differs from an *infusion* or *extract*, which pulls vitamins and volatile oils from *soft* plant material like leaves and flowers. Both decoctions and infusions have their proper place in medicine, but it's important to understand when trying to make Essiac tea that the preparation is a decoction.

Now for the good stuff: here's precisely what Essiac tea contains and how to prepare it:

— 6 1/2 cups chopped burdock root (cut into pea-sized pieces)
Burdock root has been used for many centuries and by many people as a blood-purifying herb to neutralize and eliminate poisons from the body.[4] Studies have demonstrated definitive antitumor activity in burdock root, and Japanese scientists have isolated a certain antimutation property in the plant that they refer to as "B factor."[5] The World Health Organization also recognized burdock root as being effective in the treatment of human immunodeficiency virus, or HIV.

— 1 pound powdered sheep sorrel (including the roots)
Sheep sorrel is the "mystery weed"; a retired doctor once told Nurse Caisse if everyone used it, it would result in "little or no cancer in the world." Sheep sorrel is the primary tumor-dissolving herb in Essiac tea, and it contains a unique substance known as aloe emodin that fights leukemia. Sheep Sorrel is also densely packed with a range of powerful antioxidants, or as Jon Barron of the Baseline of Health Foundation puts it, "one of the most potent antioxidant herbs known.[6]

— 1/4 cup powdered slippery elm bark
This soothing herb is a powerful anti-inflammatory that's traditionally been used to treat sore throats, diarrhea, and urinary problems. Slippery elm bark also contains a substance known as beta-sitosterol, a

plant sterol that studies have shown modulates cholesterol absorption and decreases cancer risk.[7]

— 1 ounce powdered Turkish rhubarb root
Also known as "Turkey rhubarb," Turkish rhubarb root is a staple in Traditional Chinese Medicine because it's been shown to help alleviate the symptoms associated with hypertension, menopause, gastrointestinal upset, fevers, and more. Substances like anthraquinones, tannins, calcium oxalate, and fatty acids also act as powerful anti-inflammatory and antioxidant agents, with emodin, the most highly concentrated anthraquinone in rhubarb root, demonstrating powerful anticancer potential.[8]

To properly prepare Essiac tea:

In a stainless steel pot with lid, combine 1/2 cup of the herb mixture* into one gallon of pure, unchlorinated water and boil for 10 minutes.

Turn off the heat and allow the herbs to steep for 12 hours.

After 12 hours, reheat the tea to steaming, *but not boiling*, and allow the herbs to settle for a few minutes.

Strain off the hot liquid into sterilized canning jars—you can save the leftover pulp and use it for healing poultices.

Refrigerate the tea. For long-term storage, use the boiling water bath canning method and store the tea in cool, dark, dry place.

For preventative purposes, combine one to two ounces of Essiac tea with about 1/2 cup of hot water and drink daily. Be sure to drink plenty of water (at least 1/2 gallon) daily to flush the toxins out of your system.

If you already have cancer, take this same dosage *three times* daily, and be sure not to eat or drink anything else one hour before or after the treatment. Essiac tea is compatible with most other alternative cancer treatments except for Protocel. My advice if you decide to make and start using Essiac tea is to pick up a copy of *The Essiac Book* by Mali Klein and read it in conjunction with the treatment.

*This recipe will produce 8 to 10 cups of dry herbs, which is enough to produce 16 to 20 gallons of drinkable Essiac tea. The best way to preserve extra dry mixture for later use is to put it into an airtight glass container and store it in a cool, dark place. Since the dry herb mixture is light sensitive (as is the brewed tea itself), keeping it out of direct light or in an ultraviolet-protected brown glass jar is your best option.

When using Essiac tea, also be aware that it can have a laxative effect and cause you to urinate more often than normal; this, of course, is due to its detoxifying properties. Some people report developing headaches, swollen glands, skin redness and inflammation, and flu-like systems, all of which are normal parts of the detoxification process.

HOXSEY TONIC

In Chapter 3, I gave you some background into the life of Dr. Harry Hoxsey and his famous Hoxsey Tonic, which is a lot like Essiac tea in its purpose and functionality. But I didn't give up the recipe for this tea, which I'm about to do for you now. Though Dr. Hoxsey typically customized his tea depending on a patient's particular cancer, the basic solution was standardized and included the following two ingredients: cascara sagrada (*Rhamnus purshiana*) bark powder and potassium iodide, an essential mineral that's widely regarded for supplying the body with necessary iodine, which helps support thyroid health, balance hormones (which is essential for preventing cancer!), and mitigate radioactive damage.

Other important herbs used in the traditional Hoxsey Tonic preparation include:[9]

- Poke root (*Phytolacca americana*)—10 milligrams
- Pokeweed help boost immunity, increase lymphocytes, and increase immunoglobulin.
- Burdock root (*Arctium lappa*)—10 milligrams
- Burdock root reduces mutagenicity and exhibits considerable antitumor activity.
- Barberry or berberis root bark (*Berberis vulgaris*)—10 milligrams
- Burberry contains lycbetaine, a powerful antitumor compound.
- Buckthorn bark (*Rhamnus frangula*)—20 milligrams
- Buckthorn is antileukemic and, as I mentioned earlier, contains an array of anthraquinones that are powerfully antitumoral.
- Stillingia root or Queen's Delight root (*Stillingia sylvatica*)—10 milligrams
- Stillingia is both anti-inflammatory and anesthetic.
- Prickly ash bark (*Zanthoxylum Americanum*)—5 milligrams
- Prickly ash helps improve circulation and warm the body while alleviating conditions of the stomach and digestive organs.
- Red clover blossoms (*Trifolium pratense*)—20 milligrams
- Red clover is one of the richest known sources of isoflavones, which are known to help block certain forms of cancer.

Dr. Eva Urbaniak, N.D., also includes licorice root at 20 milligrams in this same formula, as licorice root helps soften skin and mucosal membranes while quelling inflammation and relaxing muscles. Licorice root also helps support the adrenal glands and has expectorant properties that help break up congestion.[10]

I got a chance to speak with Pamela Kelsey, who not only once but twice used the Hoxsey Tonic to successfully cure cancer. The first time she did it with an aggressive form of pancreatic cancer that doctors told her was "incurable," and the second time she did it with liver cancer. Her story is an incredible one, and I'll let you hear it in her own words:

I had this horrible pain . . . I was in bed, off and on, for about a year with low blood sugar, abdominal pain, and then it got worse and worse to the point where I felt like I had a knife through the middle of my chest and out of my back.

So a friend said, "I know a friend who was cured. She had inoperable cancer of the colon and she went to a clinic in Mexico and she's five years clear of cancer." So my husband and I didn't waste any time.

We came right down to Mexico . . . I took the medicine home, the tonic, and the supplements. I was very diligent, religiously so, about sticking to the diet, doing everything the doctors told me. And within a year—well, they told me that within three months I was start to feel better—and so it was almost three months to the day that I was able to start not having so much pain.

My migraine headaches were not so frequent, not so intense. And I gradually stopped—I gradually, month by month, stopped having the pain in my abdomen. I could start digesting my food and I got better. And within a year I was clear of cancer of the pancreas.

As for the liver cancer she developed several years later, Pamela returned to the Bio Medical Center and followed the same regimen, which reduced some 22 focal lesions covering half of her liver down to just three in less than three

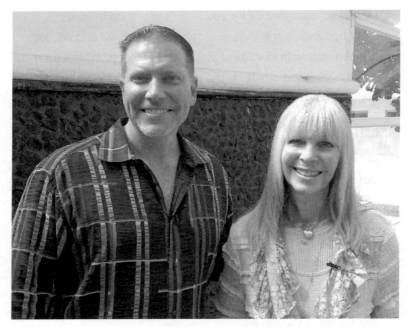

With Pamela Kelsey in Tijuana, Mexico

months. Just a few short weeks later, the remaining three lesions disappeared as well, and Pamela was declared cancer free. "I'm the longest, to my knowledge . . . living cancer survivor of the pancreas and I'm alive and well 40 years later. The doctors have confirmed that there is no longer any trace of cancer in my body. And I'm just radiant with happiness because I know that this treatment works and I know that had I done the conventional treatment I wouldn't have lived."

As with Essiac tea, taking the Hoxsey tonic can result in loose stools and possible dehydration, which in turn can lead to an electrolyte imbalance. The buckthorn and cascara components of the tea are also known to potentially deplete potassium levels, which is why it's important to consult with a qualified physician who can monitor your nutrient levels and help keep you balanced during and after treatment.

CANNABIS (HEMP)

Considered by many to be one of the most versatile healing plants in the world, *Cannabis sativa*, which also goes by names like hemp, marijuana, and "weed" depending on how it's used, is gaining a lot of attention these days on the cancer treatment front. Reports of people juicing cannabis leaves and eating high-potency cannabis oil to cure chronic diseases like cancer are everywhere, and you might be surprised to know that such medical uses are definitively backed by science.

Though it's been on the record since at least the 1970s that cannabis targets and destroys cancer cells, the U.S. government officially regards the plant as being medically useless, which is why it's still "illegal" at the federal level. Because of this longstanding policy of prohibition, research into the therapeutic potential of cannabis remains limited, though there's enough of it to suggest that serious reform is needed, and *now*.

It's a fact that cannabis has over 25,000 uses, both industrially and medically. It was grown in colonial America by some of our early presidents, and it's been used as medicine throughout the world for thousands of years. Only within the last 100 years was its reputation tarnished by special interest groups.

Now that the cat's out of the bag and people are learning that cannabis isn't the harmful vice or "devil's weed" that the drug warriors have long claimed it is, we're seeing a resurgence of interest into its therapeutic use, particularly as a treatment and *cure* for cancer.

Last year I got the chance to speak once again with Dr. Patrick Quillin, Ph.D., R.D., C.N.S., author, lecturer, and former vice president of nutrition at the Cancer Treatment Centers of America. Dr. Quillin operates his own "pharmacy" at home—think dozens upon dozens of medicinal plants that he grows in his yard, and I'll touch on them later in the diet section of this chapter—and what he told me about cannabis was intriguing.

Nutritionally speaking, hemp, which is what cannabis is typically called when we're talking about the seeds and oil sold legally in grocery stores throughout the country, is densely packed with omega-3 fatty acids, clean protein, and other vital nutrients. As I explained in my last book, hemp oil also contains up to 5 percent pure gamma linolenic acid, the highest concentration among all known plants.

These nutrients are inherently anticancer in their own right, but then you've got the host of cannabinoid compounds in cannabis that were made for the body's built-in endocannabinoid system, which is basically a communications hub in the body and brain that regulates a number of important functions, including thoughts, feelings, movements, and reactions.

Nutritional hemp products derived from "industrial" cannabis (the nonpsychoactive kind) contain only trace amounts of these healing cannabinoids, while therapeutic cannabis, which includes the kind people smoke, contains much higher levels of an anticancer substance known as tetrahydrocannabinol, or THC. THC often gets a bad rap as the "high"-producing chemical that supposedly makes people lazy while encouraging addiction. But THC is in fact a proven anticancer substance with tremendous potential to make chemotherapy and radiation *obsolete*. Dozens of scientific papers have shown that THC causes cancer cells to commit suicide. This has been seen in cancers of the brain,[11] lung,[12] bile duct,[13] skin,[14] blood,[15] and many others.

"There's quite a lot of cancers that should respond quite nicely to these cannabis agents," says Wai Liu, an oncologist from the University of London's St. George's Medical School, who coauthored a paper on the anticancer benefits of cannabis in a 2013 edition of *Anticancer Research*. Stating that cannabinoids display "potent anticancer activity" and significantly "target and switch off" certain pathways that allow cancers to grow in ways that that expensive pharmaceuticals don't, Liu added:

> If you talk about a drug company that spent billions of [dollars] trying to develop these new drugs that target these pathways, cannabis does exactly the same thing—or certain elements of cannabis compounds do exactly the same thing—so you have something that is naturally produced which impacts the same pathways that these fantastic drugs that cost billions also work on.[16]

But it doesn't stop there. Many other studies have shown that THC is medically beneficial in the treatment of ALS (Lou Gehrig's disease), Alzheimer's, anxiety, arthritis, chemotherapy side effects, Crohn's disease, chronic pain, fibromyalgia, HIV-related peripheral neuropathy,

Huntington's disease, incontinence, insomnia, multiple sclerosis, pruritus, sleep apnea, and Tourette syndrome.[17]

And then there's CBD, or cannabidiol, the nonpsychoactive component of cannabis that helps balance out the "high" feelings associated with THC. Most of THC's effects are felt above the shoulders, interacting with cannabinoid receptors type 1 (CB1), which are primarily in the brain. CBD, on the other hand, has more of a "body" effect, interacting with CB2 receptors that are more closely aligned with inflammation and related diseases.

Both substances are important therapeutically, but CBD possesses adaptogenic properties that help balance adrenals and modulate hormone production and release, particularly in response to stress. Since we know that stress is a major factor in disease, CBD in combination with THC can help give the body a break, so to speak, while also quelling inflammation and killing cancer cells.

Here's what the United Patients Group says about the benefits of CBD:

> CBD is used to help with acne, ADD, anxiety, arthritis, cancer, chronic pain, depression, diabetes, Dravet syndrome, epilepsy, glaucoma, Huntington's disease, inflammation, mood disorders, multiple sclerosis, neuropathic pain, Parkinson's schizophrenia, and neurodegenerative diseases such as Alzheimer's. CBD has also been shown to stop the spread of cancer cells.[18]

There are a number of other cannabis constituents with their own healing properties as well. These include the preheated forms THC (THCA and THCB), CBN, and CBC, among many others that I won't cover here. Suffice it to say that cannabis is a therapeutic *powerhouse*, and the sooner it's removed from Schedule I status and its prohibition is lifted, the better off the general population will be, healthwise.

"Nearly all medicines have toxic, potentially lethal effects. But marijuana is not such a substance," declared former DEA (Drug Enforcement Administration) administrative law judge Francis L. Young in response to a 1988 petition seeking to reschedule cannabis.[19] He went on to explain just how safe cannabis truly is compared to the medicines with which most people are familiar. "There is no record in the extensive medical literature describing a proven, documented cannabis-induced fatality. . . . By contrast aspirin, a commonly used, over-the-counter medicine, causes hundreds of deaths each year."

Compared to most other things people consume or take on a regular basis, Judge Young added:

> In strict medical terms marijuana is far safer than many foods we commonly consume. For example, eating ten raw potatoes can result in a toxic response. By comparison, it is physically impossible to eat enough marijuana to induce death. . . . Marijuana, in its natural form, is one of the safest therapeutically active substances known to man. By any measure of rational analysis marijuana can be safely used within a supervised routine of medical care. . . . It would be unreasonable, arbitrary, and capricious for the DEA to continue to stand between those sufferers and the benefits of this substance.

Cannabis as *food* is one way to take advantage of its healing benefits. Dr. William Courtney, founder of the Cannabis International Foundation, says THCA, the preheated, acid form of THC, can be taken at doses in the hundreds of milligrams range, as opposed to about 10 mg for high-producing THC.[20] Dr. Courtney knows firsthand the antioxidant, anti-inflammatory, and neuroprotectant benefits of THCA (tetrahydrocannabinolic acid) and its counterpart CBDA (cannabidiolic acid) because his wife, Kristen Peskuski, found relief from a number of chronic illnesses after she started taking it daily. "About four to six weeks after I started on juicing every day, I had no more back pain," the chronic sufferer of lupus, arthritis, and endometriosis explains.[21]

"Cannabis is a unique functional food [that] if used in its natural state, daily, provides benefits in excess of nutrition," adds Dr. Courtney, noting that cannabis, in his opinion, is "the most important vegetable on the planet." He recommends juicing 15 cannabis leaves and two buds daily, mixed with fruit or vegetable juice to taste.

"Cannabis provides highly digestible globular protein, which is balanced for all of the essential amino acids. Cannabis provides the ideal ratio of omega-6 to omega-3 essentially fatty acids. Critically, cannabis is the only known source of the essential cannabinoid acids. It is clear that all seven billion individuals would benefit from access to cannabis as a unique functional food."[22]

What about "pot," the kind of cannabis most of us remember from back in the '60s? Smokable cannabis buds and cannabis-derived oils have their place in functional medicine too. California was the first state in the Union to legalize medical cannabis back in 1996, and patients there have been using cannabis flowers to relieve pain, ease nausea, promote appetite, and quell anxiety, among many other uses. People used natural cannabis for such purposes long before pharmaceuticals even came into existence.

One of the most promising cannabis varietals for treating cancer is "Phoenix Tears," a rich cannabis oil developed (rediscovered) by Rick Simpson, a Canadian man who successfully used it to cure his basal cell carcinoma. Rick has been helping people in his community and throughout the world make Phoenix Tears at home, and the remedy has been such a success that many medical cannabis dispensaries now manufacture and sell Phoenix Tears directly to patients.[23]

Because of the plant's illegality in many states, raw cannabis leaves, dried cannabis buds, and oil extracts like Phoenix Tears can be difficult to come by, though there are now 24 states in the U.S. that have full medical marijuana laws currently on the books.[24] I expect that many more will join the liberty movement in the coming months and years. But we must continue to speak out so this valuable medicine can one day be removed from the prohibition list once and for all.

Cannabis oil helped save the life of Trevor Smith, who in 2012 was diagnosed with stage T2A bladder cancer. In combination with a complete dietary overhaul in which he ate *no* processed foods whatsoever and just plenty of organic chicken, vegetables, nuts, seeds, and fresh juices, Trevor successfully overcame his illness by drinking Essiac tea and taking regular doses of highly concentrated cannabis oil.

Trevor's wife, Carol, published an article about her husband's amazing journey in 2014, explaining how these natural, herb-based treatments helped him become completely cancer free, even after being told that he would never survive unless he took chemotherapy and radiation.[25] "The combination of the changing the diet, the vitamin C, vitamin D, the hemp (cannabis) oil, the vitamin B17—all of that in combination and keeping a positive mental attitude" is what cured Trevor, Carol explained to me during an interview I conducted as part of my docuseries "The Truth About Cancer: A Global Quest."

While there are no *toxic* side effects to taking either CBD or THC, THC can have mild brain effects such as anxiety and euphoria. In higher medical doses, and depending on the strain used, cannabis and cannabis extracts can also induce drowsiness, so it's important to gradually acclimate your body as you begin treatment.

DETOXIFICATION

Some level of exposure to cancer-causing chemicals is inevitable no matter how rigorous you are in maintaining a clean diet, staying hydrated, exercising, getting rest, and supplementing with anticancer "superfoods." This is why I advise everyone to *detoxify* their bodies on

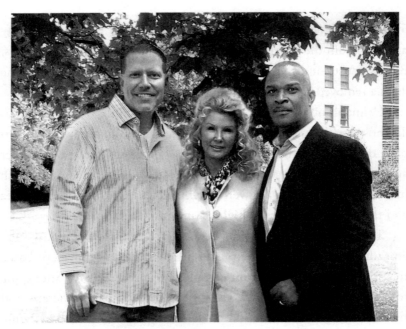

In London with Carol and Trevor Smith

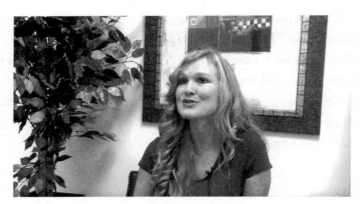

Betsy Dix

a regular basis; by this I mean a more aggressive cleansing protocol that targets specific vital organs for waste removal.

The body has its own detoxifying mechanisms such as the lymph nodes, liver, and kidneys, of course, but these organs can become overburdened depending on your level of toxic exposure. If more toxins are coming in than are being flushed out—which is pretty common in today's polluted world—the end result is decreased oxygen delivery to cells, a sluggish colon, and heightened vulnerability to bacteria, viruses, fungi, and parasites: not exactly the place you want to be.

You see, toxins lower the pH of your blood, causing it to become acidic. This creates a breeding ground for microbes, and *not* the kinds that help you digest your food. These foreign invaders are given a free pass to hijack healthy, aerobic cells and turn them into cancerous, anaerobic cells, which is where disease begins. Toxins also deplete your energy and cause your body and breath to stink, not to mention their role in causing toxemia, or the "dirtying" of your blood.

There's a process to this progressive toxification that I call the "Domino Effect," which is basically the order in which bodily organs become toxified. It all starts in the colon when a compromised intestinal lining allows toxins to "leak" into the bloodstream, where they not only pollute the blood but end up overwhelming the liver. When the liver receives more toxins than it's able to handle, these toxins are passed on to the kidneys, and then to the lymph nodes, and finally to the bladder, which is when the body has reached maximum, systemic toxicity.

"After years of research, the first exposure point that we found was the intestinal lining," Dr. Edward F. Group III, D.C., N.D., speaker, author, and CEO of the Global Healing Center explained to me about where cancer typically starts. "We figured that cancer would not exist in the body if these chemicals and toxins were not coming through the intestines and ultimately getting in the bloodstream. Once they were in the bloodstream, they went through the liver . . . and we found that everybody with cancer was completely toxic and infested, and the liver as toxic, the intestines weren't working properly, the liver wasn't functioning properly."

This is the type of scenario I don't want *anyone* to have to suffer, which is why I recommend detoxifying regularly. One physician whose entire treatment protocol focuses on detoxification of all the body's systems is Dr. Rashid Buttar. His healing protocol revolves around detoxifying from what he calls "the seven toxicities."

According to Dr. Buttar, the seven toxicities are "Heavy metals, the persistent organic pollutants, the 'opportunistics' (like bacteria, viruses, spirochetes, mycoplasma, and yeast). The fourth one is energetics like electromagnetic radiation, microwave energies, and ambient cell phone radiation. The fifth one is the most important, in my opinion, and that's the emotional psychological toxicity. The sixth one is foods . . . and the seventh toxicity is spiritual. So these toxicities that I'm talking about—that's the first step. We deal with all those things."

Betsy Dix is a patient of Dr. Buttar's who successfully used his detoxification protocol. In her own words:

I was diagnosed with cancer the first time in 2014 by an oncologist here in Charlotte, NC. It was stage II ovarian cancer. Then five and a half months later . . . I was diagnosed with this secondary primary breast cancer that was also developing at the same time, unaware to my oncologist. The conventional treatments in my case, the only conventional treatment I did was surgery. I was one of the fortunate few that had a cancer, primary cancer, and organs that were not necessary for life. I had a full hysterectomy. It did work in that it did remove the cancer, a primary portion of the cancer, and it had not spread and it was not in my lymph system yet. However it was the treatment that the oncologist wanted to do—the chemotherapy—and it was not just plain "use one port and put chemotherapy"—administer it up here. They also wanted to put a second port on my rib cage, and they wanted to do something called intraperitoneal chemo where they would have been giving me chemo, blowing out my abdomen like I'm pregnant every Monday and blowing out my veins with a second chemo. It was the over-the-top, aggressive chemotherapy they wanted to do that made me cringe. I lost twenty pounds after the surgery just thinking about the chemotherapy. I dropped to a hundred and six pounds and was in menopause and was just a mess. My oncologist was ready to put poison in my body. I was like, "I can't do this."

Then she found Dr. Buttar.

Dr. Buttar, I believe, hits cancer from many angles. You've heard or may have read his book about the seven toxicities that he mentions in his book, *The Nine Steps to Keep the Doctor Away.* I believe I had many of these toxicities. Not only was my body toxic with metals, it was also toxic with pollutants and, I also believe, emotionally and psychologically. I had gone through three miscarriages trying to conceive our second and third daughter. And during these times of grief, that really contributed, I believe, to the ovarian cancer and breast cancer diagnoses that I received that year. His treatment hits all three of these toxicities. There is chelation and many different IVs that Dr. Buttar gives that help your body get rid of toxins. And I have seen my body get rid of so many toxins through the protocol at home, which is very aggressive, as well as through the chelation in the office. . . . My blood work is of a healthy thirty-something-year-old. This is really great news. My energy, my color, all of those things, my liver, my kidneys are all functioning at a hundred percent and like a healthy individual would be.

It is important to detoxify in the proper *order*. Many medical doctors and health practitioners agree that a proper cleansing regimen is sequenced like this:

COLON CLEANSE

The bulk of your immune system—as much as 90 percent!—lives in your colon. And this is the first place where toxic waste makes its home, typically in the form of impacted fecal matter along the inner walls of your small intestinal lining: thus the popular phrase "death begins in the colon." If we are to achieve optimal health, regular colon cleansing is a must. Epigenetic Labs has an excellent colon and lymphatic cleanse product called Optimoxx, which can be found at www.epigeneticlabs.com/optimoxx. (Full disclosure: I'm a part owner of Epigenetic Labs.)

Maintaining a healthy colon is a *daily* endeavor, which is why I also recommend supplementing with a quality probiotic. There's no use in cleansing your bowel if you're not going to follow up by actually *repairing* it; "friendly" microflora are designed to populate the gut and ward off viruses, bacteria, and other pathogens, not to mention environmental toxins.

PARASITE CLEANSE

They're often an overlooked factor in the detoxification process, but parasites are arguably the most *significant* contributor to cancer among the toxins, and here's why: parasites *feed* on sugar, simple carbohydrates, and other junk food products, as well as your blood, creating the conditions necessary for cancer to flourish. Parasites also feed on mycotoxins like aflatoxin, which grow as mold on food.

"Make no mistake about it," Dr. Hazel Parcells once stated, "worms are the most toxic agents in the human body. They are one of the primary underlying causes of disease and are the most basic cause of a compromised immune system."

In order to effectively rid your body of parasites *and their eggs*, you need the following three things:

- Black walnut hulls (from the black walnut tree)
- Wormwood (from the artemisia shrub)
- Cloves (from the clove tree)

The black walnut hulls and wormwood will kill both the adult and developmental-stage varieties of more than 100 known parasites, while the cloves will kill the eggs. Artemisinin, a compound in wormwood, is also an effective inhibitor of angiogenesis, cutting off the blood supply of cancer tumors so they can't survive.

As an aside, another effective way to minimize your exposure to mycotoxins is to wash your food with ozonated water, which helps neutralize them as well as kill parasite eggs and other invaders.

KIDNEY CLEANSE

Your kidneys are the filtration system for your blood, which is why performing a kidney cleanse is next on the list. Together, the kidneys filter up to 150 quarts of blood *daily*, producing up to two quarts of urine waste. When toxins build up and begin to overload the kidneys, kidney stones can begin to form—and in a worst-case scenario, the kidneys can shut down altogether.

For daily kidney maintenance, you can eat large amounts of watermelon and drink celery seed tea. For a more aggressive cleanse, you can follow the kidney/liver cleanse product formulated by Dr. Daniel Nuzum and available at www.epigeneticlabs.com/optimoxx/.

LIVER/GALLBLADDER CLEANSE

Next we have the liver and gallbladder, which also filter blood and aggressively target bacteria and viruses. The liver regenerates itself every six weeks; it's that important! But when it becomes compromised, symptoms often aren't noticeable. When the liver is healthy, there's almost *no* disease that can overtake the body. This should tell you a lot about the state of most people's livers!

Here's an easy liver and gallbladder cleansing protocol that you can do at home with simple ingredients:

- Drink one quart of organic, unprocessed apple juice every day for three days. Apple juice is rich in malic acid, which acts as a solvent to break up adhesions and soften liver and gallbladder waste globules for elimination.
- On the evening of the third day, drink eight ounces of organic, cold-pressed, extra virgin olive oil. Stir with the juice of one lemon and drink it down quickly.
- Lie down on your right side in the fetal position for 30 minutes, keeping a small trash can nearby in case you experience nausea-induced vomiting, a possible side effect of this cleanse.
- The next morning when you have your first bowel movement, you should see small black and green pebble-like pieces in your stool; these are gallstones!

Another very effective method of detoxifying the liver is by utilizing a coffee enema. Believe it or not, coffee enemas were included in *The Merck Manual* until the 1970s as the most effective method to detoxify the liver. Also, Dr. Daniel Nuzum has developed an amazing liver/kidney cleanse product available at www.epigeneticlabs.com/optimoxx/.

BLOOD CLEANSE

When too much toxic waste enters the bloodstream due to gut leakage, veins and arteries begin to lose their elasticity and harden. Inorganic waste material builds up on the inner walls of the circulatory system, weakening its functionality. Blood purification is absolutely essential to keep this "river of life" flowing and delivering nutrients and oxygen.

An herbal cleansing tonic made from many of the same ingredients found in Hoxsey tea, Essiac tea, and a formula developed by Dr. Richard Schulze—red clover, burdock root, chaparral, poke root, and sheep sorrel—will do the trick. Jon Barron also sells an herbal tincture that, depending on your level of toxicity, can be taken at doses between 4 and 12 droppers-full daily.[26]

He's become something of a legend in the natural health world: Jared Bucey, the famous "Kid Against Chemo," who, after suffering in misery and almost dying as a result of chemotherapy, opted for alternative remedies instead. Jared homed in on detoxification as his cancer weapon of choice, and as he told me personally, it was the right decision—he now lives a vibrant, cancer-free life. Jared explained:

I didn't really know too much about cancer or chemo, and I didn't think there [was] much of a cure for cancer. I thought cancer pretty much is my death right on the spot. . . . I did one round, one full cycle of chemo and then all the side effects were just so severe. I had really bad mouth sores throughout my whole GI system. I had really bad bone pain. I couldn't stand. I couldn't walk. My parents had to help me walk to the bathroom and back. I could barely use my phone or the TV remote because my hands were cramping from the bone pain.

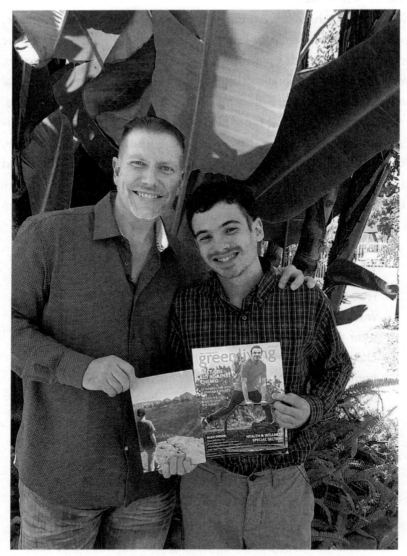

With Jared ("Kid Against Chemo") in San Diego

Jared knew that the chemotherapy was harming him, but his doctors were insistent that he continue it anyway. They even resorted to overblown fear tactics by claiming that if Jared didn't run the full chemotherapy course, he would die a slow, painful death that felt like drowning.

But being the smart young man that he is, Jared did his own research and opted to go down a different path that ultimately proved his doctors wrong, while also saving his life! "I just do all alternative methods from vitamins, supplements, infrared sauna, all organic juice, and all raw vegetables," he told me about how he overcame his diagnosis. Jared is now healthier than ever before!

Again, when initiating any detoxification protocol, be aware that your body will be going through immense changes that may provoke various elimination and "die-off" symptoms. These may include headaches, fever, upset stomach, diarrhea, skin breakouts, and other uncomfortable but common side effects.

GERSON THERAPY

It's important to keep in mind that any detoxification protocol is only as effective as its conjunctive nutrition protocol, which is why the most efficacious therapeutic approaches include both for comprehensive healing. The Gerson Therapy is a great example of this philosophy, combining the power of aggressive cleansing with high-density nourishment to maximize the body's intrinsic ability to heal itself of chronic disease.

Originally developed in the 1930s by the late Dr. Max Gerson as a natural remedy for his own chronic migraines, the Gerson Therapy is used today to treat everything from skin tuberculosis and diabetes to autoimmune disorders and cancer. It's an all-encompassing body replenishment protocol that addresses the two primary causes of degenerative disease—toxicity and nutrient deficiency—hence its incredible, nonspecific ability to tackle a vast array of health issues.

The Gerson Institute explains:

> The Gerson Therapy is a natural treatment that activates the body's extraordinary ability to heal itself through an organic, plant-based diet, raw juices, coffee enemas and natural supplements. The Gerson Therapy regenerates the body to health, supporting each important metabolic requirement by flooding the body with nutrients from about 15–20 pounds of organically grown fruits and vegetables daily. Most is used to make fresh raw juice, up to one glass every hour, up to 13 times per day. Raw and cooked solid foods are generously consumed. Oxygenation is usually more than doubled, as oxygen deficiency in the blood contributes to many degenerative diseases.
>
> The metabolism is also stimulated through the addition of thyroid, potassium and other supplements, and by avoiding heavy animal fats, excess protein, sodium and other toxins.

The Gerson Therapy also utilizes intensive detoxification to eliminate waste buildup, regenerate the liver (your body's main detoxifier), boost the immune system, and restore the three key systems that make up the body's natural defense arsenal—the enzyme, mineral, and hormonal systems: "With generous, high-quality nutrition, increased oxygen availability, detoxification, and improved metabolism, the cells—and the body—can regenerate, become healthy and prevent future illness."

There are currently two inpatient facilities where patients can receive Gerson Therapy under the guidance and supervision of a qualified physician and trained staff: the Gerson Clinic in Tijuana, Mexico,[27] and the Gerson Health Centre in Budapest, Hungary.[28]

The Gerson Institute has also provided free information online for individuals looking to administer the Gerson Therapy at home with the help of friends and family members.[29]

I've had the privilege of meeting a number of individuals over the years who successfully overcame what many doctors claim are untreatable chronic illnesses using Gerson Therapy. One such individual is Dr. Felicity Corbin-Wheeler of London, a British Red Cross nurse who told me about her amazing recovery from pancreatic cancer using Gerson Therapy.

Dr. Corbin-Wheeler has an extensive background in the medical field, having worked for one of London's top cancer surgeons, and is well versed in the politics of modern medicine. She's also painfully familiar with the devastating effects of cancer, having had several of her family members—including her own daughter—die from it. After eventually being diagnosed herself with pancreatic cancer, which she believes to be the consequence of many years of drinking chemical-tainted well water on her family's farm, Dr. Corbin-Wheeler began to venture down the conventional treatment route—that is, until a pastor at her church, a former gastroenterology nurse, told her about another way.

"Behold, I have given you every plant yielding seed that is on the surface of all the earth, and every tree which has fruit yielding seed; it shall be food for you": these are the precious words from Genesis 1:29–30 that would forever change Dr. Corbin-Wheeler's life, leading her to vitamin B17 (laetrile from fruit seeds) and Gerson Therapy.

"I was laying there in agony, being sick and feeling really dreadful, thinking, 'I think this is probably right. We've got to detox.' I then did lots of research. I got onto the Gerson Therapy. I got B-17 from Mexico from Dr. Francisco Contreras," she explained to me. "And I got well."

DIET FOR LIFE

Sometimes reversing cancer is as simple as changing one's diet, which is why I want to emphasize once again the importance of *nutrition* in overcoming chronic disease. Your body continually regenerates itself based on the "fuel" you give it, and if you're constantly pumping diesel into the tank when unleaded gasoline is what you need, you're going to have a rough ride and eventually experience a breakdown.

There are as many dietary protocols for cancer as there are stars in the sky, it seems. But I'd like to focus on the foundational principles that weave a common thread through all of them. Everything you put in your body either *fuels* cancer or *deters* it. I'll try to make things clearer for you by breaking it all down into these two categories.

Cancer-*fueling* foods are those that lower pH and are nutritionally deficient, tainted with toxins, and conducive to cancer cell growth. These include things like refined sugar, processed flour, trans fats, MSG, nitrites, aspartame, conventional products, and really anything that's been highly processed and has a long list of ingredients; such foods are typically found on shelves in the *inner* aisles of the grocery store.

Cancer-*fighting* foods are those that help balance pH and kill cancer cells, and nearly all of them are dense in vitamins, minerals, and enzymes, which I covered earlier. These include things like organic produce, grass-fed and pasture-raised meats and dairy products, cruciferous vegetables (broccoli, cauliflower, and brussels sprouts), nuts and seeds, saturated fats, herbs, and clean, mineral-rich water.

Some specific cancer-fighting foods, herbs, and nutrients that I'd like to highlight include:

Turmeric (curcumin). This cancer-fighting herb of the highest order is capable of repairing damaged DNA, protecting against xenoestrogens (which often cause cancer), destroying free radicals, and even preserving delicate nutrients in food. One of the most potent antioxidants known to man, turmeric is virtually unmatched in its detoxifying, cancer-fighting, and anti-inflammatory potential.[30] An excellent product that contains three different types of fermented turmeric along with vitamin D3, ashwagandha, and ginger is called Turmeric 3D and can be found at https://epigeneticlabs.com/turmeric-3d/.

Apple cider vinegar (ACV). Made from fermented apple cider, ACV has been used since the time of Hippocrates to treat indigestion, pneumonia, scurvy, and various other illnesses. ACV is an amazing detoxifying and purifying food rich in antiseptic and antibiotic amino acids. ACV is an excellent addition to your daily detoxifying regimen, helping dissolve mucus and phlegm deposits; cleanse the kidneys, liver, and bladder; and oxygenate and thin the blood for improved flow.[31]

Enzymes. I mentioned earlier that without enzymes, even the healthiest foods on the planet are near useless. You need protease enzymes to digest protein, amylase enzymes to digest carbohydrates, and lipase enzymes to digest fat. Unfortunately, many foods these days are lacking in enzymes, which is why most people should probably supplement with them to keep things functioning.

A few great options that I'd recommend are Vitälzym Cardio by World Nutrition Inc.,[32] VeganZyme by the Global Healing Center,[33] and Wobenzym N by Garden of Life.[34]

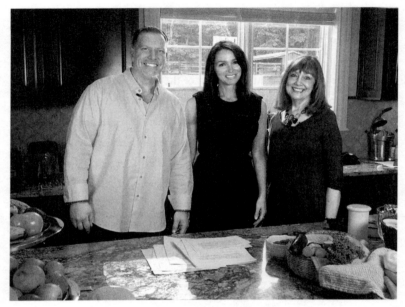

Ty and Charlene with Cherie Calbom

Raw juices. Fresh juice from a press is naturally high in enzymes, and if you can find fruits and vegetables grown in *biodynamic* soils without chemical pesticides and herbicides, it's also high in easily assimilable nutrients. My family and I like to juice carrots, celery, cucumbers, beets, and apples, and we'll often add ginger, parsley, and other healing herbs to taste. I interviewed Cherie Calbom (aka "The Juice Lady") last year, and she recounted an amazing story when she first began juicing. In her own words: "So I decided to do a five-day juice fast. On day number five, this is honest truth, my body expelled a tumor the size of a golf ball. About that big, with blue blood vessels attached to it. Looked like somebody just chopped them off. And that got my attention, like nothing else."

One of the most amazing—and surprisingly tasty—juices is wheatgrass juice. It's one of the most oxygenating superfoods in existence due to its high chlorophyll content. Wheatgrass is also rich in selenium and laetrile, the same substance found in peach pits that's used at the Oasis of Hope Hospital to treat cancer.[35]

Medicinal mushrooms. Mushrooms have been treasured as both medicine and food for thousands of years. Most medicinal mushrooms contain polysaccharides (complex sugar molecules) called "glucans" that increase DNA and RNA in the bone marrow, where immune cells (like macrophages and T-cells) are made. Reishi mushrooms have been used as a medicine in Asia for over 4,000 years, and the Japanese government officially recognizes reishi as a cancer treatment. In China, a maitake mushroom extract was shown to have an anticancer effect in patients with stomach cancer, lung cancer, and leukemia. In Japan, clinical studies have been conducted on lentinan (a glucan), found in shiitake. These studies have shown that treatment of advanced-cancer patients with intravenous lentinan results in increased number and activity of immune killer cells and in prolonged survival. A seven-year study funded by the National Institutes of Health and reported in

November 2010 found that the use of turkey tail mushroom significantly boosted immunity in women who had been treated for breast cancer. An excellent supplement that contains seven different types of fermented medicinal mushrooms is called 7M+ and can be found at https://epigeneticlabs.com/7m-plus/.

Fermented and sprouted foods. By definition, sprouts are edible plant seeds that have begun the germination process—meaning they're beginning to grow into mature plants. Like other vegetable foods, sprouts can vary in texture and taste. Perhaps you're acquainted with hardy bean sprouts (small, light yellow leaves and silvery white shoots) or threadlike alfalfa sprouts (thin, delicate, and green), which are readily available at your local supermarket or health food store. The soaking process is the catalyst to turning these seeds into tiny nutritional powerhouses with readily bioavailable vitamins, minerals, and proteins plus beneficial enzymes and phytochemicals. Sprouting occurs in nature through germination, which is the way the plant brings food forth from the soil. This process breaks down the natural agents (known as antinutrients) in the seed's outer coating that protect the seeds from early germination and predators. One of these antinutrients is phytic acid, which can do a number on your digestive system.

Besides sprouting, another way to unleash the power of nature in your diet is through the process of fermentation: the culturing or natural souring of foods through the intentional growth of bacteria, yeast, fungi, or mold. It's a time-honored method that allows foods to stay edible longer. For most of recorded history, fruits, vegetables, dairy, and meats had no "shelf life" unless you put them through a fermentation process. Preservation of vegetables and fruits by fermentation has numerous advantages beyond those of simple shelf life extension. During fermentation, starches, sugars, and proteins in vegetables and fruits are converted into organic acids—such as acetic and lactic acid—by the many species of bacteria, yeast, and fungi.

This transformation of normal foods into superfoods makes them more nutritious and easier to digest and assimilate. What history's indigenous cultures have long known about fermentation is becoming increasingly studied, tested, and accepted in today's world of science.

Saturated fats. Saturated fats haven't exactly been given a fair shake over the last half century. Health authorities basically lumped them in with trans fats when it came to their supposed negative impact on health. But saturated fats like those found in coconut oil, butter, ghee, and lard are food for the brain, and they're also a necessary building block for hormone production.

Saturated fats also facilitate nerve communication in the regulation of metabolism and insulin release. Coconut oil, one of the healthiest forms of saturated fat and a rich source of medium-chain fatty acids, is an appetite stimulant that helps boost energy levels and promote weight loss. The lauric acid in coconut is especially beneficial in fighting off pathogens, yeast (candida), and molds, which makes it a great addition to the above detoxification protocols.

And don't forget fish oil, avocados, and extra virgin olive oil. Though none of these are saturated, each one represents an important fat for health and vitality:

- Fish oil is a rich source of the omega-3 fatty acids EPA (eicosapentaenoic acid) and DHA (docosahexaenoic acid), which are converted into hormone-like substances called prostaglandins that impact cardiovascular health and regulate cell activity.
- Extra virgin olive oil is full of antioxidants and its monounsaturated fatty acids help balance cholesterol levels.
- Avocados contain high levels of oleic acid, which helps protect against breast cancer. They also contain lutein, tocopherols, and

the carotenoids zeaxanthin, alpha-carotene, and beta-carotene, which help protect against prostate cancer.

WHAT YOU NEED TO KNOW

- Prevention is the best approach to dealing with cancer and other chronic diseases, and prevention is best achieved by minimizing exposure to toxins; eating a clean diet; exercising (and sweating!) regularly; minimizing stress; and maintaining healthy relationships.
- If you're already suffering from chronic disease, high-potency herbal protocols like Essiac tea, Hoxsey Tonic, and cannabis can provide relief, especially when combined with an aggressive detoxification protocol.
- Chronic disease is typically a factor of two things: toxic buildup and nutrient deficiency. Protocols like the Gerson Therapy bring both areas back into alignment by ridding the body of what's keeping it sick and building it back up with aggressive nutrient intake.
- The most important thing of all is *diet*, which includes intake of both high-nutrient foods and supplements (preferably whole-food-based, unless otherwise administered under the supervision of a qualified physician).

CHAPTER 10

SOUND, LIGHT, ELECTRICITY, FREQUENCY, AND HEAT

The only thing that really differentiates the "alternative" cancer treatments to which I'm introducing you from the "conventional" methods with which most people are familiar is their recognized *status*: the former aren't officially "approved" by government authorities and the latter are considered by these same authorities to be the *only* way to effectively treat cancer—that and the fact that these alternative methods actually *work* without damaging your cellular system and DNA, which can't be said for chemotherapy or radiation.

I've never really liked the word *alternative* in reference to functional medicine because this disparaging descriptor makes it sound as if there's one solid standard contrasted by *everything else*, when in reality "alternative" medicine was the accepted standard long before what's now considered to be conventional medicine even came into existence. This disparity between what we're told is true—that conventional medicine is science-based medicine—and what's *actually* true has made some people very wealthy, but it's done serious damage to public health. And it's cost many people their *lives*.

Setting the record straight and helping you avoid the trap that is conventional medicine are the reasons I'm writing this book, and I feel privileged to have your attention on these important matters. What I'm about to unveil to you about the power of sound, light, and *energy*, and how these material functions of our universe are uniquely equipped to heal, will probably blow your mind. I know it did mine when I first heard about it, yet it's been right in front of us—and all around us!—since the beginning of time.

In ancient mythology, Apollo, the Greco-Roman god of medicine and healing, rode his "fiery chariot," the sun, across the skies every day, bringing both light and warming energy to the world. As the story goes, the sun's energy was recognized as having the power both to harm and to heal, and from a healing perspective we can now see, based on modern science, that there's more than a grain of truth to this ancient myth.[1]

For at least the past century, the primary focus among health professionals has been on the supposed harm caused by sun exposure, harm that sound science would contend is a factor of one's ability to properly receive the sun's energy. Let me put it another way: if your body and skin are lacking in antioxidants, you're far more likely to be *burned* by the sun than energized by its vitamin D–producing rays.

There's a common theme here that I feel the need to stress over and over again in order for it to sink in. It's the very thing Louis Pasteur admitted on his deathbed about the nature of disease: that the pathogen is nothing, and the terrain is everything. Except in this case, we're talking about energy rather than pathogens—energy that, given the proper terrain, acts as *healing* rather than harming energy, particularly in the realm of cancer.

THE HEALING POWER OF "ENERGY" MEDICINE

So-called "energy" medicine can mean a lot of things. On the metaphysical end of the spectrum, it can typify a spiritual healing approach that involves things like touch, energy points, chakras, auras, and other so-called New Age concepts. On the other end of the spectrum is a more tangible use of the forces of energy: think therapies that utilize light, heat, and even sound to achieve a certain health outcome.

Conceptually speaking, this particular type of energy medicine utilizes many of the same technologies used in traditional diagnostics: things like PET (positive emission tomography) scans, MRIs, CT scans, ultrasounds, and the like. These methods are generally accepted as useful when it comes to *diagnosing* a health condition (using energy to look for malignancies and malfunctions in the body) but for some reason they're not yet accepted as *treatments* for health conditions.

It's unfortunate, really, because these methods, as you're about to learn, are both powerful and effective. They've been in use at clinics throughout the world for many decades, including at the renowned Hope4Cancer Institute in Baja California, Mexico. The clinic utilizes a combination of light (photodynamic) and sound (sonodynamic) therapies to treat cancer patients. Depending on the type of cancer, one or the other, or both, therapies are employed for maximum effect. "Our general strategy is to intensively treat the areas where cancer is present or is likely to be present with the semilocal PDT (photodynamic therapy) and SDT (sonodynamic therapy), and the whole body with less intense systemic PDT," the clinic explains on its website.[2]

I got the chance to sit down with Dr. Antonio Jimenez, M.D., founder and medical director of the Hope4Cancer Institute, and he explained to me in detail how the process works. In a nutshell, a special sensitizing agent is administered to cancer patients, and this agent acts as a type of Trojan horse to gain entry into cancer cells. Once inside,

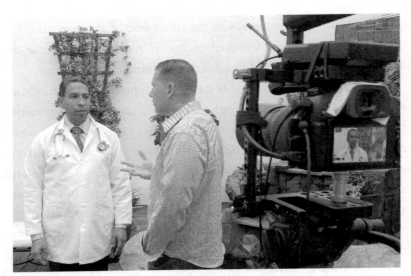

Filming with Dr. Antonio Jimenez in Tijuana, Mexico

this agent awaits its "orders" from either light or sound, or both, to release an oxygen molecule that effectively kills the cell on contact.

This sensitizer, Dr. Jimenez explained to me, has an almost universal propensity for malignant cells, with only a very small number of healthy cells getting caught in the fray. And those few healthy cells that absorb the sensitizer spit it out within a day or two, which is how the Hope4Cancer Institute team knows when it's time to administer the treatment. Since the type of sensitizer Dr. Jimenez and his colleagues use is naturally occurring and completely nontoxic (the chlorophyll derivative of seaweed), patients can rest assured that they aren't being systematically poisoned with a toxic chemical in the process of being treated for their cancers.

"We provide what's called a sensitizer and the patient takes this under the tongue, based on his body weight," Dr. Jimenez explained to me. "This (sensitizer) is absorbed by cancer cells seventy to one. So, for every seventy cancer cells, one normal cell absorbs this molecule. . . . We wait twenty-four to thirty-six hours after administration (to begin treatment). This way, most of the cancer cells have now all absorbed it and normal cells have released it."

Dr. Jimenez knows the treatment works because his clinic has had an incredible rate of success treating patients with it. But he's also a humble man who openly admitted to me that the mechanism behind *why* it works remains a mystery: "I think it's a God thing, but, you know, that's another story."

We do know this much, though: the sensitizing agent used at the Hope4Cancer Institute, which goes by the name of "SP-Activate," is positively charged. As it turns out, cancer cells, which are *anaerobic* in nature as opposed to *aerobic* like healthy cells, are drawn to this positively charged substance.

So of what, exactly, do Dr. Jimenez's treatments actually consist? The clinic uses both sound and light energy to trigger SP-Activate within the body. The sound component utilizes specific frequencies, amplitudes, and intensities to "wake up" the sensitizer so it will activate itself within cancer cells, producing oxygen radicals. Also known as "O-minus" radicals, these oxygen molecules initiate apoptosis, or programmed cell death.

The light therapy component performs much the same function, using a system of lights—red, blue, and "invisible" lights on the near infrared spectrum—to activate the sensitizer and kill cancer cells. This process also produces localized inflammation to heighten the body's immune response, which aids in this eradication of cancer cells. "This is full spectrum light," Dr. Jimenez emphasized. "There is no mercury being released here. This is not fluorescent light . . . the closest we can come to mimicking the light of the sun. And you know, from historical records, we know that the sun has healed many diseases."

SP-Activate works best against superficial cancers like those of the prostate, breast, and skin, which are the easiest to access with light, sound, and lasers. But it also works well against deep tumors and systemic cancers like those of the bowel and ovaries when *heat* is added to the mix, a method known as hyperthermia sono-photo dynamic therapy.

Photodynamic therapy is used both systemically and semilocally at the Hope4Cancer Institute. Patients are typically instructed to lie down in a special machine, face down, for 30-minute sessions, during which time their bodies are exposed to the full spectrum of therapeutic light. Large areas of the body can be effectively treated in this manner because the entire body is essentially receiving the treatment.

Sonodynamic therapy is very similar in that it uses a variety of sound frequencies as a semilocal therapy to treat various cancers. The sounds used have been carefully fine-tuned for maximum reception by SP-Activate, which makes this method highly effective as well. The clinic prefers to use *both* therapies for optimal benefits, and research shows that utilizing both sound and light acts as a one-two punch against cancer.

I touched on this earlier, but for the SP-Activate to actually work, it must have access to oxygen in order to kill the cancer cell that it's occupying. This is where a hyperbaric oxygen chamber comes into play. "What this does is the patient comes in here, lies down—and it's very comfortable—and we increase the pressure of oxygen to between four and four point five pounds per square inch," Dr. Jimenez explained as he showed me the machine in person at his clinic. "We know oxygen and cancer don't combine. And so, the one hour that the patient is in here, you're saturating the cells with oxygen."

The normal amount of pressure, I soon found out, is about 1.3, which means a hyperbaric oxygen chamber applies about *four times* as much pressure as normal, delivering much more oxygen to the cells for maximum effect. Patients apparently love the feeling of being inside the chamber because they can actually *feel* the oxygen making its way into their bodies, strengthening and rejuvenating their faculties. "Some patients ask me, 'Can I stay in here two hours or three hours?' Literally you could, because you can't get too much oxygen in this sense, but one hour is the duration of the treatment."

As I learned about the sequence from start to finish, I was fascinated by the duality of how simple and straightforward it is: light, sound, and oxygen are apparently all you need to kill most cancers! All the tools we need to cure cancer are right in front of our eyes, and the work being done at the Hope4Cancer Institute is a perfect embodiment of this.

Trina Hammack, a health care practitioner from California, told me all about her experience at the Hope4Cancer Institute when she was treated for stage IV ovarian cancer. She opted out of chemotherapy and radiation treatments and

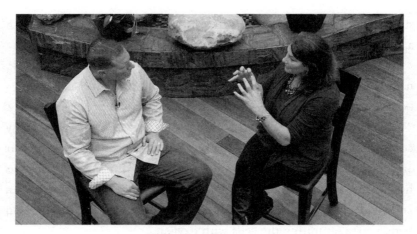

With Trina Hammack

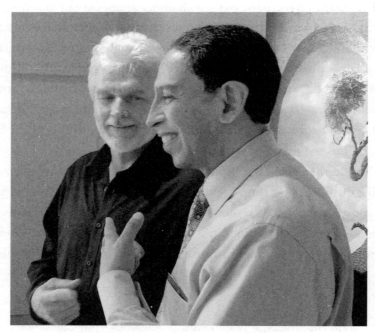

Dr Tony Jimenez with Charles Daniel

decided to undergo sono-photo dynamic therapy (SPDT) under the guidance of Dr. Jimenez, who she's been referring her own patients to for many years. "Dr. Tony was my hope because I knew him and I've known him for years and I'd seen the success [when] I'd send my clients," she recalled to me during an interview.

After undergoing a pelvic exam and getting a blood test done, it was confirmed: Trina had a melon-size tumor in her ovaries that a combination of surgery and SPDT would effectively treat. "I began the Sono-Photo treatments and during the first few weeks watched my CA-125 (a tumor marker) plummet. All of my doctors were monitoring my lab reports and CT scans, and with each report the news was better and better. Soon the cancer was completely gone!"[3]

Charles Daniel has a similar success story with invasive cancer of the bladder. He was supposed to have had a 90 percent chance of being cured with surgery alone, until doctors realized that the cancer had aggressively spread to both his lymph nodes and liver. At the behest of his oncologists, Charles soldiered through a subsequent round of chemotherapy, which eliminated two of his three liver tumors and significantly shrunk the third. This was then followed up with another post-treatment surgery and a round of infusions and nutritional supplements, which Charles hoped would cure him once and for all.

When the cancer came back with a vengeance, Charles underwent yet *another* surgery to have the new tumor removed, but was told he was no longer eligible for chemotherapy: his body simply couldn't handle it. Desperate for a solution, Charles, his wife, and his brother and sister-in-law began researching alternative options and eventually came across the Hope4Cancer Institute. "I came to Hope4Cancer, completed the inpatient program, and continued the home program, and I'm happy and proud to say that since that time, all of my tests and scans have indicated that I'm cancer free," Charles explained during an interview.[4] "My oncologist told me that the average life expectancy for someone with bladder cancer in the liver was nine months, and he had never seen anyone go past twelve months. I feel like Hope4Cancer gave me a second chance at life. . . . The treatments at Hope4Cancer were nontoxic, I didn't have any adverse side effects, and to me the treatments were easy."

ELECTROMAGNETIC ENERGY: IS IT ALL BAD?

Normally when we speak of electromagnetic frequencies, it's in a negative light. This is because EMFs, or so-called "dirty electricity," are considered harmful radiation, the kind that propels off a cell phone tower to your mobile phone and into your ear (and brain!), or from your television or microwave into your body. This kind of pollution is highly damaging to your cells, both healthy and malignant alike.

But there's another kind of electromagnetic energy that's actually *beneficial*: *pulsed* electromagnetic fields, or PEMF. This type of electromagnetic energy has been scientifically shown to have a positive effect on the body when used properly.

PEMF is used at the Hope4Cancer Institute to treat cancer, but it's been in use for much longer than that by an unlikely entity: *planet Earth*. The earth, as you probably know, has its own magnetic field that's constantly moving and changing due to heat convection radiating out from its inner core. As the earth spins on its axis and around the sun, this field generates constant forces that are crucial for maintaining the life-forms we see all around us, including humanity itself.

Without this magnetic field, *we wouldn't be alive*. It's a reality that the first astronauts experienced during the early days of space travel when they suffered from what we now refer to as "space sickness." Soviet cosmonaut Yuri Gagarin made history when he was the first to orbit the earth for a nearly two-hour space flight, during which time he became very ill. Gagarin had everything his launch crew thought he needed—air, food, water, light, and limited movement—but they forgot one thing: electromagnetic energy. Once this invisible force was understood as an essential component for life, every astronaut after Gagarin was accompanied by special PEMF devices during flight.

Why is PEMF so important? Well, for starters, the entire functionality of the cellular system is dependent upon it. Uptake of oxygen, cellular energy production (ATP), nutrient assimilation, waste removal, enzyme activity: everything your body needs to live comes to a screeching halt when this vital source of energy is missing. And one of the "symptoms" of the damage caused by this lack of energy is—you guessed it!—cancer.

Our bodies were made to harness energy, you see, but they only do so when the proper energy receptors are in place. These substances, which we refer to as electrolytes, are ionically charged when properly positioned throughout the body. They act as energy *conductors* to capture and utilize magnetic field energy, in the process fueling our cells and organs to do their respective jobs.

"The body is electric," says Dr. William Pawluk, M.D., an expert in magnetic field energy who's been featured on *The Dr. Oz Show*.[5] "The water in a human body (or other terrestrial creature) is not unlike the electrolyte solution in a battery. It is composed of many electrolytes, along with saline. . . . Electrolytes compose both positively and negatively metallic ions, including sodium, potassium, calcium, chloride, etc. . . . Magnetic fields cause or increase motion of ions and electrolytes in the tissues and fluids of the body. This movement stimulates a vast array of chemical, mechanical, and electric actions in the tissues of the body."

Because of a lack of nutrition, environmental pollution, and various other factors, many people's bodies have become ill equipped to capture and use magnetic field energy, which is why PEMF therapy is becoming so popular. Resulting poor cell membrane performance is now considered by those in the know to be one of, if not *the*, leading cause—or at the very least, co-factor—in the development of chronic and autoimmune diseases.

According to Nobel Prize winner Otto Warburg, every cell in your body has what's known as transmembrane potential, or TMP, which is basically an energy marker of that cell's ability to produce ATP, which you'll remember from earlier chapters is the energy currency of your cells' mitochondria. A normal TMP falls somewhere between 70 and 90 millivolts, but this number can drop due to age, sickness, environmental chemicals, and even stress.[6]

A TMP of around 50 millivolts will make a person feel tired, and possibly chronically fatigued. How many people do you know these days who suffer from perpetual sleepiness? Perhaps you're one of them! But it gets worse. If TMP voltage drops to between 15 and 30 millivolts, cells are extremely likely to become cancerous.

Remember, when cells' ATP production is lagging, their ability to accept and deliver oxygen quickly follows suit. This is about the time when aerobic cells begin to switch to anaerobic cells to accommodate their changing environment, and before you know it, a full-blown tumor starts growing and metastasizing.

Getting these cells back on track is the purpose of PEMF therapy, which helps jump-start cellular voltages back to where they need to be for optimal cellular function. It's a lot like jumping a car with a dead battery, giving it the "kick" it needs to start running on its own.

"Therapeutic magnetic fields are used to induce voltages similar to those produced naturally within the body at the cellular and subcellular level," adds Dr. Pawluk. "The electromagnetically-induced field accomplishes the result of transferring charge to cells of the body. This induced current can lead to nerve firing, muscle contraction, stimulation of cell signal pathways causing cell growth, and a number of other effects. Because of this most basic level of treatment, magnetic therapies have been shown to have positive effects in a myriad of conditions."

From a cancer perspective, PEMF helps raise the overall TMP of the cellular matrix in order to weed out and fix the cancer cells. When these damaged cells become properly "charged," they rather quickly revert to their normal aerobic states and begin producing ATP, accepting oxygen, and moving electrolytes and other nutrients in and out of the cellular system as needed.

"PEMF research proves routine neurological, physiological, and psychological repair," says holistic lifestyle researcher and educator Marcel Wolfe. "When the frequency is spot-on, absolutely nothing compares—not far infrared, not laser, not ultrasound. PEMF research has repeatedly proven better physiological repair in far less time than any other type of care while indicating absolutely no adverse reactions."

The American Institute of Physics published a paper in 2007 revealing that Dr. Pawluk, Wolfe, and many others are absolutely right about the benefits of this unique therapy. Electric energy fields most certainly *do* disrupt the division and spread of cancer cells, and have been shown to effectively slow the growth of brain tumors in human clinical trials.[7]

FREQUENCY GENERATORS THAT KILL CANCER

In an earlier chapter, I gave you a little background on the work and legacy of Dr. Royal Raymond Rife, who was one of the groundbreaking pioneers in modern-day frequency therapeutics. Similar in concept to PEMF therapy, high-radio-frequency generators based on those first developed by Dr. Rife are being used today in energy medicine, and you can actually purchase them for use at home.

These high-RF generators are designed to match the unique electronic signatures of the pathogens that live inside malignant cells in order to trigger their self-destruction, which in turn causes them to destroy the malignant cells in which they were living. As with PEMF, there is no actual destruction of cancer cells taking place, at least not directly; high-RF generators target the parasitic elements living *within* cancer cells so that they'll turn on their hosts.

By killing their pathogenic invaders, high-RF generators allow cancer cells to revert to their normal, precancerous state. It's almost as if these matching frequencies cause damaged cells to come to the sudden realization that they've been going down the wrong path, prompting them to quickly turn around and start supporting the body rather than continuing to destroy it. "When Dr. Rife was able to kill the virus and/or bacteria [that was] inside of a cancer cell, the cancer cell was able to restore its metabolism and become a normal cell (i.e. 'revert' into a normal cell)," writes Webster Kehr for the Independent Cancer Research Foundation, Inc. "Let me say that again a different way: It is possible to kill the microbes which are inside of the cancer cells, which allows the cancer cells to restore their metabolism and thus revert into normal cells."[8]

It's a highly efficient way to eradicate cancer cells without harming healthy ones, and without having to go to extreme lengths to do so. Killing the microbes that are causing the damage in the first place also kills cancer cells, and the immune system regenerates. And these high-RF frequency machines can be used in conjunction with anti-cancer nutritional protocols like the Cellect-Budwig protocol[9] and the Plasma-Beck protocol.[10]

In fact, it is probably *best* that they be combined with a solid nutrition regimen because, as I keep saying, diet is the most important part of the equation when it comes to preventing and treating cancer.

IS YOUR WATER ENERGY ACTIVATED?

In the aftermath of the great Chernobyl nuclear disaster of 1986, a Russian scientist named Dr. Igor Smirnov was asked by the Soviet government to conduct an assessment of cancer rates in the area. He was tasked with looking specifically at a small subset of people who, unlike the 3 million or so fellow countrymen who had developed cancer from the radioactive fallout, were mysteriously healthy and cancer free.

You've probably never heard much about what he found, but I got the chance to interview Dr. Howard Fisher, D.C., an antiaging expert and best-selling author from Toronto, Canada, who worked alongside Dr. Smirnov, and he told me that the secret was in the water. Flowing from the Caucasus Mountains are "supercharged" water molecules that possess an unprecedented ability to hydrate cells, Dr. Fisher explained to me, and people living near Chernobyl who drank this water in the 1980s developed a type of protection against radioactive poisoning. "If you can super hydrate a cell, i.e., if you can get enough water into the cell so it functions optimally, it can basically take on almost anything," Dr. Fisher told me about the amazing healing power of this "high-energy" water.

"What was happening was the structure of this water was changing by coming over the Caucasus Mountains and instead of being isotetrahedral or pyramidal, it was coming in a linear format . . . access[ing]

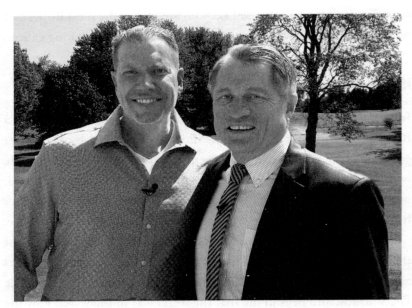

With Dr. Howard Fisher in Toronto, Canada

something called aquaporins [that] go into every cell, carry nutrition into every cell, (and) bring toxins out of every cell."

Once it was understood that the molecular structure of this water is different from that of other types of water, Dr. Smirnov and those who discovered it got to thinking: What if everyday water could be molecularly altered to provide the same healing benefits to people who don't live near the Caucasus Mountains? This is how Molecular Resonance Effect Technology, or MRET, came into existence.

A proprietary, patented noise field technology that generates a subtle, low-frequency energy field very closely resembling the natural geomagnetic field found near healing water springs, MRET activates and changes the molecular structure of water into a highly intelligent, bioavailable form that helps revitalize the body and enhance its ability to function.[11]

Your cells actually prefer the type of energetically charged spring and mineral water that rolls off the sides of pristine mountains and flows through many layers of lava rocks because this type of water is the most efficient at hydrating and powering the cellular system. This water isn't a *cure* per se for cancer, but its effect on the physiological functionality of your cells enables them to target and destroy cancer on their own.

Dr. Peter Agre was awarded a Nobel Prize in 2003 for discovering the presence of aquaporins in healing water, which are essentially integral membrane proteins that effectively channel water molecules across cell membranes and into the cells. Aquaporins are *essential* for cell hydration, and hydration is the means by which cells protect against pathogenic invasion and resultant disease.[12] "Viruses in a dehydrated cell can multiply easily," says Dr. Fisher, illustrating this point.

MRET water is designed to mimic the effects of energy-charged spring water, helping hydrate cells three times faster than ordinary water can. MRET water also promotes improved cellular and circulatory function, better cell communication, balanced intestinal flora, and perhaps most importantly of all in light of this book, optimized anticancer abilities.

There are no chemicals or foreign substances involved in the process of making MRET water, and anyone can do it at home using a simple MRET water activator system.[13] It's really a great option for staying both hydrated and oxygenated.

HYPERTHERMIA AND THE POWER OF HEAT

And last but not least in the healing energy category: the *heat* factor. You're probably already familiar with what happens when you contract a serious illness and your body goes into hyperdrive by reacting with a fever, or high temperature. This hyperthermic response is the body's way of naturally fighting the infection, and contrary to popular belief, it shouldn't be minimized with ibuprofen and other drugs because it's a *good* thing, despite being uncomfortable.

As it turns out, hyperthermia is also beneficial in the treatment of cancer. In 1893, Dr. William B. Coley discovered how the body's hyperthermic response to bacteria can also help kill cancer cells. He purposely injected bacterial toxins into the tumors of 10 cancer patients and watched as their bodies responded with fevers, effectively killing the tumors.

A later study from Germany replicated this by demonstrating that Coley's toxins, which are now referred to as mixed bacterial vaccine (MBV), helped cure advanced-stage non-Hodgkin lymphoma, resulting in a 93 percent remission rate as opposed to a dismal 29 percent remission rate among controls who received chemotherapy, and such research is continuing.[14]

The use of induced hyperthermia in anticancer therapeutics is a rapidly expanding field, yet its effective application has been around for more than 100 years. In 1927, Julius Wagner-Jauregg was awarded a Nobel Prize for his work in hyperthermic therapies, but how many people do you know today who are utilizing it in the fight against cancer?

It's a shame, really, because hyperthermia is a highly effective way to kill cancer cells. They only need to be heated to about 108 degrees Fahrenheit for roughly one hour in order to die. Healthy cells, on the other hand, die at a much higher temperature, so this heating process is completely safe and 100 percent selective, destroying *only* malignant cells.

Even better is the fact that this gentle heat promotes blood vessel dilation around healthy cells, *improving* their function—this while knocking out cancer cells with ease. Because cancer tumors are tightly packed with very little circulation, heating them in order to kill them just makes logical sense. And microwave energy is one powerful way to do this, as cancer tumors have a high water content.

The beauty of microwave energy, as Dr. Alan J. Fenn, an electrical engineer at the Massachusetts Institute of Technology, found throughout his research, is that it's adaptive. This means it can be concentrated directly into a tumor without harming other tissues, which seems to be a pattern among alternative cancer therapeutics.[15]

But there are many other ways to induce hyperthermia, including fullbody submersion into hot water, ultrasound, and one particular modality that seems to be growing in popularity at an accelerating rate: infrared saunas. Infrared energy penetrates the skin and pulls out toxins while simultaneously heating the body's internals. And depending on which end of the infrared spectrum is used—near, mid, or far—heat energy can have varying beneficial effects. Here's what renowned oncologist Dr. Josef Issels, once stated about the power of heat: "Artificially induced fever has the greatest potential in the treatment of many diseases, including cancer."[16]

This is quite the powerful statement—and by a cancer doctor, no less! But it's true, and there are several important reasons why. First, hyperthermia helps eliminate from the body lingering toxins that contribute to cancer. Hyperthermia also helps improve circulation, improving the flow of oxygen to cells while flushing acidic waste from their structures. And finally, hyperthermia kills cancer cells on contact by heating them to a temperature beyond what they can handle.

Some cancer clinics utilize hyperthermia machines like the BSD-2000 Hyperthermia System in conjunction with traditional therapies like chemotherapy and radiation. One example is the BSD Medical Corporation based in Salt Lake City, Utah, which obtained a Humanitarian Use Device to use with the BSD-2000 in the treatment of cervical carcinoma.

I'm of the persuasion that there are much better ways to utilize hyperthermia *without* tying it in with radiation and poison. But unfortunately for Americans, it's difficult to find such treatment options without going overseas to places like China and Germany where innovative approaches to its use are welcomed rather than scorned. I will say that hyperthermia is by no means a stand-alone treatment for cancer because it doesn't possess the ability to boost immune function, a key component of the healing process. The only way it can is by combining it with a powerful nutrition program.

The Hope4Cancer Institute recommends adhering to a customized, holistic nutrition program that centers around things like getting the proper amounts of macronutrients and micronutrients. This can involve juicing, fermenting, and sprouting nutrient-dense foods, as well as making sure that you're getting plenty of antioxidants, whole-foods based vitamins and minerals, complex carbohydrates, protein, healthy fats, and of course, clean water.

My good friend Enoch DeBus, a certified nutritionist and cancer survivor, told me recently about how he combined heat *and* nutrition into a single protocol he used to keep himself free of cancer. Many spices and hot peppers contain compounds such as capsaicin that help raise body temperature naturally, creating an internal "sauna" factor that wards off disease. "I've got a variety of ingredients that I use," he explained to me about his "Kick 'Em Juice" health tonic. "I've got ginger, and I try to use everything organic . . . ginger, turmeric . . . [and] I'll take the hottest peppers I can find—habaneros, cherry peppers, jalapeños—the hottest ones that are available that are in good shape. I'll take those, chop them all up, and I'll take my ginger and brew it for about thirty minutes. I'll bring it to a boil, let it simmer for around thirty minutes, then I'll drop in my hot peppers for another ten minutes. And then . . . I'll put some raw ginger, some raw turmeric, put it in, and I'll put it in a blender."

Enoch says he's always had an extreme sensitivity to environmental pollutants, and learned very early in his life how to take advantage of nature for his own benefit. This knowledge came in handy later on in adulthood when Enoch was involved in a serious car accident that left him stricken with severe gastrointestinal problems. He was told he would have to have his gallbladder and appendix removed so doctors could "explore" the area further, something he declined in favor of a heating cleanse.

"I didn't do anything but drink that master cleanse, which is lemon or lime, with organic maple syrup, about a tenth of a teaspoon per serving of cayenne powder. And then in the morning, you take that throughout the day; I'd drink about twelve glasses of it a day while I was working. It kept my energy up great."

Enoch also used his Kick 'Em Juice to treat a basal cell carcinoma he developed not long after that. Once again

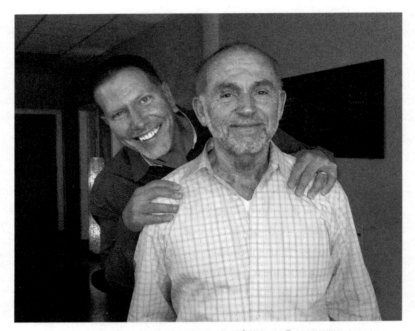

With Enoch DeBus in Atlanta, Georgia

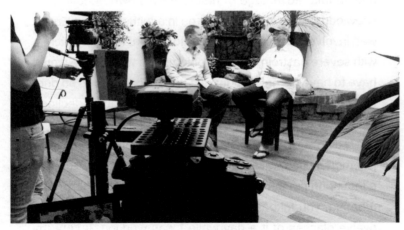

With Michael Stephenson

avoiding invasive surgery, Enoch took the juice, and within a matter of days began to experience relief. "This Kick 'Em Juice is what I felt the Holy Spirit inspired me to make and the bleeding stopped within days," he told me, adding that his cancer was completely *gone* about a month later.

Michael Stephenson is another cancer conqueror I spoke with who was cured of prostate cancer using a different kind of heat therapy. After going around in circles with oncologists who wanted to randomly blast his prostate area with radiation even though his prostate had already been removed in a previous surgery—the surgery failed to eradicate the cancer, it turns out—Michael decided to fly down to the Hope4Cancer Institute in Tijuana, where he was subjected to the "pig cooker," a heat chamber where he sweated for 45 minutes.

Michael also did coffee enemas to clean out his bowel, as well as an "antivenom" therapy whereby his own urine was used as a type of inoculation to rid his body of PSA. Dr. Jimenez and his colleagues taught Michael and his wife some therapies to do at home as well that would "supercharge" his body, and this combination of therapies did the trick.

"When I went home, I built my own (infrared sauna) in my garage, and heated that sucker up to 140 degrees," Michael told me, obviously thrilled about how heat therapy had helped him so immensely.

I'll leave you with this final quote from Parmenides, the famous Greek physician who more than 2,000 years ago demonstrated a solid understanding of heat therapy and its importance in warding off disease: "Give me a chance to create fever, and I will cure any disease."[17]

WHAT YOU NEED TO KNOW

- Energy is a critical component of the healing process, coming not only from food but also from light and even sound. Energy from the sun, for instance, enters the skin in the form of ultraviolet rays and produces immune-boosting vitamin D. And the antioxidants in nutrient-dense foods help protect your skin so you don't "burn" during this energy transfer.
- Various photodynamic (light-based) and sonodynamic (sound-based) therapies can help oxygenate cells and promote cellular health, preventing otherwise healthy cells (aerobic) from going rogue (anaerobic).
- Pulsed electromagnetic frequencies (PEMF) are also beneficial when applied properly, promoting cell oxygenation, cellular energy production, nutrient assimilation, and enzyme activity, all processes that maintain homeostasis in the body.
- The human body is made mostly of water, and this water functions as a system of vibrational energy. When health problems arise due to vibrational failure, frequencies can be used to bring it back into alignment.
- Heat is beneficial to health, helping to destroy pathogens and even cancer cells while preserving friendly microflora and healthy cells. Both external heat (infrared saunas) and internal heat (hot peppers) confer health benefits when applied properly.

CHAPTER 11

BIO-OXIDATIVE THERAPIES

You're probably intimately familiar with the word *carcinogen* at this point, and recognize it to mean a substance that causes cancer. But have you ever thought about *why* a carcinogen causes cancer? What makes it so inherently cancer forming that simple exposure to it causes healthy, aerobic cells to switch over to an unhealthy, anaerobic state? The simple answer is that it all comes down to *oxygen*.

Oxygen is the lifeblood of the cellular system; without it, there would be no *you*. And a carcinogen, according to Otto Warburg, is any substance that deprives cells of the oxygen they need to create energy, expel waste, and perform other cellular functions essential to life.

Warburg spent many a day in his laboratory researching cytochromes and the role they play in cellular respiration. He began to notice a distinct pattern that led him to conclude that all sorts of substances are carcinogens, the common thread being that *every single one* of them impedes cellular uptake of oxygen. Recognizing that oxygen is pretty much the only substance whose absence would kill us in a matter of *minutes*, Warburg came to the conclusion that "cancer has only one prime cause. The prime cause of cancer is the replacement of normal oxygen respiration of body cells by an anaerobic cell respiration."[1]

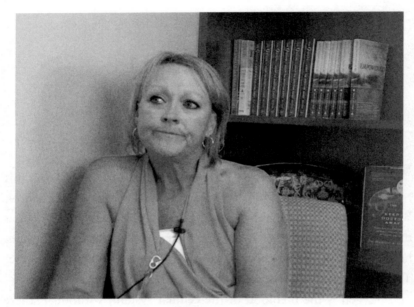

Tina Baird

It's a pretty simple concept—almost *too* simple when you really think about it—yet it makes perfect sense. When our cells have the appropriate amount of oxygen they need, cancer doesn't stand a chance. However, when they don't, we call this phenomenon *hypoxia*, and the only remedy is to bring that oxygen back through oxidative therapy.

According to Dr. Rashid Buttar, "Where growth stops, decay steps in. And so, to me, this is not a static process. Either you're getting worse or you're getting better. There's no such thing as staying right there in the middle. So physiological optimization, when you're dealing with a cancer patient would be, for example, the use of oxygen. Oxygen is highly detrimental to cancer because cancer is an obligate anaerobic metabolizer. It likes an oxygen-free environment. So if you give oxygen, it's detrimental to the cancer."

Tina Baird was diagnosed with stage 2A breast cancer in 2010. After undergoing chemotherapy, radiation, and surgery, Tina remembers thinking, *I just want to close my eyes, and I just don't want to wake up.* She was hardly eating, sick, and had lost all desire to live. Then she heard about Dr. Buttar's clinic in North Carolina. After detoxification and utilizing bio-oxidative therapy, she's alive to tell her story and healthy. As she put it in her own words, "I feel better today than I have in probably ten years. I have tons more energy."

WHY OXIDATION IS IMPORTANT FOR HEALTH

When you hear the word *oxidation*, you probably think free radical damage, a.k.a. cell damage. But oxidation is really just the interaction of oxygen with some other substance. It can be a bad thing or a good thing, depending on the substance involved. Every time you take a breath, you're oxidizing your blood and cells via your lungs, which is obviously a *good* thing. Oxidization is also how your body fends off bacteria, yeast, viruses, and parasites: the more oxygen in your cells, the more impenetrable they are to foreign invaders. It's really that simple, and it's precisely why staying oxidized is so important for your health.

I explained in the last chapter how the Hope4Cancer Institute uses hyperbaric chambers at its clinic to deliver therapeutic doses of oxygen to patients undergoing cancer treatment. This is one great option, as are "bio-oxidative therapies," which encompass an entire field of therapeutics focused on delivering two key substances to the body: hydrogen peroxide (H_2O_2) and ozone (O_3).

These two substances have been extensively documented in the scientific literature for their role in treating many of the most common diseases people face, including heart disease, AIDS, and cancer. The philosophy behind how they work, as outlined by Dr. Charles H. Farr, one of the fathers of bio-oxidative medicine who was nominated for the Nobel Prize in Medicine in 1993, is quite simple:

If there's not enough oxygen being delivered to cells, whether due to poor diet, environmental pollution, lack of exercise, or some other factor, the body won't be able to effectively eliminate toxins (bacteria, viruses, chemicals, etc.), resulting in disease. Bio-oxidative therapies fill this gap by providing the body with active forms of oxygen, whether orally, intravenously, or transdermally, so it can eliminate toxins and ward off disease.

So what do hydrogen peroxide and ozone have to do with oxygen? Once these substances are inside the body, they break down into what are known as oxygen "subspecies" that seek out anaerobic viruses and microbes—anaerobic, remember, means they survive without oxygen—as well as diseased or deficient cell tissue, and oxidize them. You can think of hydrogen peroxide and ozone as jumper cables going all around the parking lot jump-starting cars with dead batteries.

Except they're *smart* jumper cables that intuitively know which cars have dead batteries and which ones don't before they try to jump them. They *only* target the "dead" ones so as not to damage the "alive" ones (if this analogy is in any way helpful for your understanding of the process). Oxygenating anaerobic cells basically brings them back from the dead, so to speak; it roots out any lingering toxins and essentially creates a whole new cell.

For me, there's an analogy here, spiritually speaking, where what was once dead (oxygen-deprived cancer cells) has now been made alive (oxygen-saturated healthy cells). I think of it in terms of a miraculous *rebirth*, and perhaps you can relate.

OZONE: SUPERCHARGED "ACTIVATED" OXYGEN

First discovered by German-Swiss chemist Christian Friedrich Schönbein, ozone is a "supercharged" form of oxygen that contains an extra atom; a typical oxygen molecule contains two oxygen atoms (O_2), while ozone contains three (O_3). This extra atom breaks off from the other two after about 20 to 30 minutes inside the body and performs a unique function beyond just oxygenating cells.

Decoupled from their parent ozone molecules, these oxygen "singlets" are free to bind to anything and everything they can, which is good news for one's health. Viruses, bacteria, fungi, parasites, molds, and cancer cells absolutely *hate* ozone, just like they hate oxygen. So when you have free-roaming O_2 along with the O singlet roving the body, disease simply doesn't stand a chance.

As I explained in my last book, these oxygen singlets bind with other compounds like carbon monoxide (CO), which is harmful to the body, to form carbon *dioxide* (CO_2), which is beneficial. Together with the remaining oxygen (O_2) molecules, these singlets seek out and destroy any viruses, bacteria, yeast, and abnormal tissue cells they find in the body by blasting through their protective membranes, which quickly leads to their death. It's the same technique that was used in Germany during the 1930s when patients were being successfully cured of inflammatory bowel disease, ulcerative colitis, Crohn's disease, and other gastrointestinal-related illnesses.

"Ozone therapy disrupts the integrity of the bacterial cell envelope through oxidation of the phospholipids and lipoproteins," explains a clinical review of ozone therapy published in the *Journal of Natural Science, Biology and Medicine*.[2] "In fungi, O_3 inhibits cell growth at certain stages. With viruses, the O_3 damages the viral capsid and upsets the reproductive cycle by disrupting the virus-to-cell contact with peroxidation. The weak enzyme coatings on cells which make them vulnerable to invasion by viruses make them susceptible to oxidation and elimination from the body, which then replaces them with healthy cells."

In addition to going after microbial pathogens, ozone therapy also improves cell function. O_3 increases the rate of red blood cell glycolysis in the body, which in turn promotes a greater release of oxygen to cell tissue. When this happens, ATP production gets a boost as well, as does the production of important enzymes that act as free radical scavengers and cell wall protectors. These include the "master" antioxidant glutathione peroxidase, catalase, and superoxide dismutase, as well as a prostacyclin, a vasodilator.

Clinical trials involving ozone therapy have shown that the treatment reduces oxidative stress in the body; deactivates viruses like HIV; boosts immunity; and eradicates bacterial infections, all of which are directly associated with causing cancer. Ozone therapy is also used to treat chronic pain resulting from nerve injuries. So how is ozone therapy administered? There are three ways:

- *Ozone IV*: fluid saturated with ozone is injected directly into the bloodstream
- *Autohemotherapy*: 10 to 15 milliliters of blood is drawn from the body, saturated with ozone, and injected back into the body
- *Ozone sauna*: the body is enveloped with warm, humid steam to open up the pores for ozone to enter through the skin into the bloodstream

Ozone IVs and autohemotherapy are obviously the most invasive because they involve needles and blood, which for some people is a turn-off. An ozone sauna, on the other hand, is by far the simplest and most home-friendly method of getting ozone, and the good news is it's also the most effective!

There are a couple reasons for this: 1) ozone sauna therapy exposes the entire body to ozone through its largest and most encompassing organ, the skin; and 2) ozone saunas have the added benefit of applying heat to the body, which, as we previously covered, provides hyperthermic benefits. Together, ozone therapy and hyperthermia penetrate deep within tissue to oxygenate the blood and cells, draw out toxins, and improve cellular function.

"Using the steam sauna with ozone allows the steam to surround the body and ozone can be introduced through the skin," explains one source about how the ozone sauna works. "Humid heat opens the pores, which allows the ozone through the skin to the bloodstream, where it can travel to the fat and lymph tissue. It is very important to cleanse the lymph tissue of toxins and the ozone/steam sauna is the easiest and best way to accomplish this."[3]

Many people don't know this, but Dr. John Harvey Kellogg, inventor of Kellogg's Corn Flakes and the name behind the Kellogg's cereal brand, was actually a medical doctor and surgeon who embraced a naturopathic worldview. He served as editor of the *Health Reformer* journal for nearly 70 years and advocated for many of the healing protocols I've outlined in this book.[4]

Dr. Kellogg also had a thing or two to say about ozone therapy, having used it himself in the steam cabinets at his naturopathic sanitarium in Battle Creek, Michigan, the place where Kellogg's cereals are still made to this very day. In his book *Diphtheria: Its Causes, Prevention, and Proper Treatment*, published in 1880, Dr. Kellogg wrote, "Probably, no agent . . . for the purpose of purifying the air of the sick-room . . . is so useful for this purpose as ozone, one of the most powerful disinfectants known."[5]

Renowned scientist and inventor Nikola Tesla took his own liking to ozone, having developed the world's first ozone generator in 1896. In 1900, he introduced an ozone-infused olive oil that he sold to doctors for medical use. And for the next several decades before pharmaceuticals came on the scene, ozone was used to treat everything from anemia and asthma to hay fever, gout, diabetes, insomnia, pneumonia, and a whole slew of different cancers.[6]

A 1904 volume published by chemist Charles Marchand entitled *The Medical Uses of Hydrozone [ozonated water] and Glycozone [ozonated olive oil]* is still available at the Library of Congress in Washington, D.C., having been approved by the U.S. Surgeon General. A patent for ozone-infused essential oils filed by Dr. William D. Neel in 1909 is still on the books as well.

What makes ozone so special, in my view, is the way it merely catalyzes the delivery of oxygen, and ultimately *energy*, into the cells. Ozone stimulates the production of cytokines, or "messenger cells," that set off a domino effect of positive energy changes throughout the immune system, delivering more oxygen to cells so they can perform the metabolic and detoxifying functions for which they're designed.

And ozone does all this *without harming healthy cells*—how cool is that? The defensive enzymes like superoxide dismutase and glutathione peroxidase that are generated from ozone help protect healthy cells from being invaded and destroyed during the purge. It reminds me of the Passover story where the Israelites painted lamb's blood over their doorposts as protection from the plagues of God's judgment: ozone gives healthy cells the special protection they need before it comes rumbling through to ravage all the bacteria, viruses, and cancer cells polluting the body.

The unique way in which our bodies utilize ozone for health demonstrates an amazing profundity and a fascinating creativity by our Creator. I'm simply blown away by how perfectly and beautifully oxygen, in its various iterations, performs maintenance on our bodies, *especially* in the area of cancer.

Check out what this 1980 study published in the journal *Science* revealed about ozone's selective targeting of cancer cells, even when ozone is simply present in the ambient air: "The growth of human cancer cells from lung, breast and uterine cancers was selectively inhibited in a dose-dependent manner by ozone at 0.3 to 0.8 parts per million of ozone in ambient air during eight days of culture. . . . The presence of ozone at 0.3 to 0.5 parts per million inhibited cancer cell growth at 40 and 60 percent respectively."

Here's the real kicker: "Exposure to ozone at 0.8 parts per million inhibited cancer cell growth more than 90% and control cell growth less than 50%. Evidently the mechanisms for defense against ozone damage are impaired in human cancer cells."[7]

Did you catch that? Cancer cells *hate* ozone and quite literally die in its presence. Healthy cells, on the other hand, are not only immune to ozone damage, but are actually *enriched* by its presence.

While ozone is recognized by both the Environmental Protection Agency and the Food and Drug Administration as having the ability to purify water at a rate of up to 99.99 percent, its use as a therapy in medicine is limited, at least in the U.S. Ozone therapy is widely administered in Germany, where more than 7,000 currently practicing doctors have been trained in how to treat patients with it. But like most of the other alternative therapies I've covered here, testing of ozone therapy in the U.S. is forbidden.

However, there *are* clinics across the country that offer ozone therapy to patients, and ozone saunas are also available for folks who prefer to treat themselves in the comfort of their own homes, without persecution from the medical system.

HYDROGEN PEROXIDE: THE LIFEBLOOD OF THE IMMUNE SYSTEM

Proper immune function is also dependent upon the other piece of the oxygen puzzle, hydrogen peroxide (H_2O_2). Hydrogen peroxide is a key component of colostrum, an antibody-rich secretion found in breast milk, and it's also the immune system's first line of defense against infection.

Dr. Charles H. Farr, M.D., Ph.D., who's considered the "father of oxidative medicine," was a strong advocate of hydrogen peroxide therapeutics, which he claimed produces a positive metabolic effect when injected intravenously. The idea is that, much like ozone, hydrogen peroxide has a unique ability to oxidize almost any physiologic or pathologic substance, as well as produce increased tissue and cellular oxygen tensions.

He wrote that hydrogen peroxide "is produced by all cells of the body for many different physiological reasons," which is true. He also wrote that it's "involved in many metabolic pathways which utilize oxidases . . . and hydrogen peroxide is involved in protein, carbohydrate, fat metabolism, immunity, vitamin and mineral metabolism, or any other system you might wish to explore." He even went so far as to call hydrogen peroxide the "Master Regulating Molecule" of the body.[8]

A later report published in the *Proceedings of the International Conference on Bio-Oxidative Medicine* explains further how hydrogen peroxide increases metabolic rate, dilates small artery vessels for increased blood flow, eliminates toxins, raises body temperature, enhances the body's distribution and consumption of oxygen, and stimulates the production of white blood cells, which the body uses to fight infection.[9]

You're probably familiar with those 3 percent solutions of hydrogen peroxide that you can buy for a few bucks from the drug store as a disinfectant for wounds. Many people keep this type of hydrogen peroxide in their medicine cabinets as an inexpensive but effective topical cleansing solution. But you may not be as familiar with food-grade hydrogen peroxide solutions that range between 30 and 35 percent concentration; these are the kinds of hydrogen peroxide used in systemic therapeutics.

Dr. Farr preferred to inject this highly potent form of hydrogen peroxide into his patients, but others including Dr. Reginald Holman added it in small amounts to drinking water with positive success. Tests conducted in the 1950s found that cancerous rats given water containing just a few drops of food-grade hydrogen peroxide saw their tumors completely dissolve in as little as two weeks.

Diffusing hydrogen peroxide in a vaporizer is another common way to capture the benefits of hydrogen peroxide without a needle. Dr. Kurt Donsbach from the Santa Monica–based Donsbach Clinic wrote in a paper for *Alternatives*:

"One ounce of 35% hydrogen peroxide (per gallon of water) in a vaporizer every night in an emphysemic's bedroom, and they will breathe freer than they have breathed in years! I do this for my lung cancer patients."[10]

If you've ever used 3 percent hydrogen peroxide solution to treat a cut or other abrasion, you probably noticed that, upon coming into contact with the wound, the solution began to bubble up and create foam. When hydrogen peroxide encounters the enzyme catalase, which is constantly circulating in the blood, it triggers a chemical reaction that produces both water and oxygen gas—oxygen that your body uses to clean up damaged cells and essentially heal the wound!

This is pretty much the same process that occurs internally when hydrogen peroxide is present in the blood in therapeutic amounts; cells get a rigorous oxygen bath, damaged cell tissue is removed, and healthy cells become reinvigorated. The body makes its own hydrogen peroxide to accomplish these tasks, of course, but like any other nutrient, it can become depleted due to a variety of factors. Hence the need for direct intervention with either injection or oral supplementation.

The general consensus seems to be that intravenous hydrogen per-oxide therapy is the safest and most effective way to utilize this powerful substance as a healing agent. One popular method involves adding a very *weak*, pure form of hydrogen peroxide—around 0.0375 percent or lower in concentration—to a sugar or saltwater solution, and slowly injecting it at doses of between 50 and 500 milliliters over the course of between one and three hours, depending on the condition being treated.

This type of IV drip is usually administered once a week for most chronic illnesses, but it can also be given daily if a patient is suffering from something more serious like HIV/AIDS or cancer. A qualified physician will be able to make a proper assessment of what you need for your particular malady, which brings me to my next point: IV hydrogen peroxide therapy *isn't* something you should try at home, and should only be administered by a health professional who can carefully monitor your progress.

And the only kind of hydrogen peroxide you should ever take internally is the 35 percent food-grade kind, because anything else is potentially *toxic* when consumed. Just be sure that if you do take hydro-gen peroxide internally on your own, you take *small* amounts—just a few drops diluted in water—because too much can have a damaging effect on the stomach lining, especially if you're adhering to a special regimen like the Budwig diet that involves eating lots of fats.

There's also a product currently under development, named Oxycyclene, that might turn out to be an even more effective way to deliver hydrogen peroxide to the body without having to inject or drink it. It works by essentially forcing white blood cells to produce more hydrogen peroxide in order to draw out toxins and regenerate cell tissue. The Health and Wellness Foundation explains:

> The chemical principal is the selective induction of high levels of reactive oxygen species ("ROS") (superoxides/peroxides/singlet oxygen) in infected macrophages (white cells that ingest foreign matter and invaders) and dysplastic cells (rapidly proliferating tumorous macrophage cells that couldn't handle the invaders. Oxycyclene chemicals are highly concentrated (1000x greater than in normal cells) into intracellular infected cells and those that have become dysplastic from long term ROS incompetence. Oxycyclene chemicals bypass the toxin blockade to forcibly stimulate the ROS.[11]

HIGH-DOSE VITAMIN C INJECTIONS

Prior to his death in 1994, two-time Nobel Prize winner Linus Pauling made some incredible contributions to the field of science. One of these hinged upon his famous work dealing with vitamin C, which he realized could be injected intravenously at very high amounts to treat chronic illness.

Along with Dr. Ewan Cameron, an experimental psychiatrist from Scotland, Pauling developed an extensive treatise on nutritional vitamin C and how it can be used to treat everything from the common cold to cancer. Entitled *Cancer and Vitamin C*, the work is part of what made Pauling famous, along with the more than 1,000 articles and books he published during his amazing life.

One of the specific things Pauling uncovered about vitamin C is the fact that it's a *pro-oxidant*, meaning it has the ability to generate oxygenating compounds like hydrogen peroxide inside the cells. This finding was just one of *many* that comprise the field of orthomolecular medicine, to which he was a leading contributor. High-dose vitamin C therapeutics is a hallmark of Pauling's work, and for good reason: vitamin C is one of the easiest and most powerful ways to jump-start the oxygenating process in cells, and it's completely nontoxic. Here's what one of his colleagues, Dr. William Wassell, M.D., wrote about its benefits:[12] "Vitamin C is thought to act as a pro-oxidant inside the cell in high concentration, and some hydrogen peroxide is formed which is rapidly disposed of by catalase in a normal cell. Since cancer cells have a deficiency or lack entirely of catalase the peroxides kill the [cancer] cell."

The late Dr. Hugh Riordan, another one of the "fathers" of high-dose vitamin C research, was among the first to show that vitamin C can be used as an effective antitumor therapy. The key, he found, was getting high enough amounts of it into the bloodstream at one time in order to provoke the desired effect.

The reason why *injecting* vitamin C is so important, he and his colleagues found, is because oral dosages of vitamin C simply aren't high enough to have any formidable impact on tumors. Sure, you can scarf down all the vitamin C you want, but your body will only process so much of it at a time. If you take 30 to 180 milligrams per day, the absorption rate will be between 70 and 90 percent. If you take 1,000 milligrams or more per day, the absorption rate drops to about 50 percent. And it gets progressively worse the more you try to take.[13]

Vitamin C delivered through an IV bypasses the digestive tract and goes straight into the blood at a near-total absorption rate. To put things into perspective, you would have to take upwards of 1,000 to 2,000 milligrams of vitamin C orally *every ten minutes* during your waking hours of the day to even come close to the amount you would get from a single IV drip—and in extreme disease cases, the dosage could even translate to *twice* that amount. It's enough to make your head spin, and that's why IV vitamin C is the best route to take if you have cancer or some other chronic illness requiring rapid and frequent oxygenation.

Most forms of vitamin C that people take orally are water soluble, meaning any excesses of the vitamin that aren't metabolized end up getting flushed out of the body via the urine. Many forms of injectable vitamin C, including sodium ascorbate, are also water soluble, but their absorption rate via the blood, as I mentioned earlier, is significantly higher: a 2001 study found that IV vitamin C is highly toxic to cancer cells, especially when combined with alpha-lipoic acid.[14]

But there are also fat-soluble analogues of vitamin C like phenyl ascorbate that are even more potent. Studies have found that they're as effective as water soluble forms of vitamin C like sodium ascorbate, but *at one-third the dose.* This makes phenyl ascorbate an even more promising option in high-dose vitamin C therapeutics.

As science has uncovered the nuances of vitamin C and how the body absorbs and uses it, novel approaches like pulsed intravenous vitamin C, or PIVC, are gaining popularity. This method builds upon the concepts laid out by Joseph Casciari and his colleagues at the Riordan Clinic in Wichita, Kansas, where high-dose IV vitamin C therapy is a hallmark of patient care. But PIVC takes this treatment to a whole new level. Here's how the Colorado Integrative Medical Center in Denver explained its functionality:

The concept of PIVC is to get acute blood levels of vitamin C as high as possible. By simple diffusion physiology, an acute doubling or tripling of the blood vitamin C levels will temporarily allow an acute doubling or tripling of the amount of vitamin C that normally diffuses into perfused tissues via the gradient that is present at the baselines concentration.

The temporary blood levels achieved can be substantial. If Casciari et al. can get a certain high blood level from infusing 60,000 mg of vitamin C over 80 minutes, than an IV push of 20,000 mg of vitamin C over 2 minutes can be expected to temporarily increase the peak blood concentration by 10-fold or more over the rapid intravenous infusion. This amount has already been administered safely on multiple occasions.[15]

Because high-dose vitamin C injections tend to provoke a strong inflammatory response, cancer patients at risk of complications should opt for a modified treatment plan. Under the supervision of a qualified physician, a "build-up" approach will help mitigate inflammation and swelling, and help ensure a positive outcome.

UV BLOOD IRRADIATION

When a plant is exposed to sunlight, the chlorophyll inside it captures the sun's energy and combines it with carbon dioxide to produce sugar. After using what it needs, the plant then releases oxygen as "waste," which we humans and the rest of the animal kingdom take in as breath and life. It's a beautiful, codependent relationship that underpins yet another novel oxygenating treatment known as ultraviolet blood irradiation, which builds upon this concept utilizing a process known as photoluminescence to oxygenate the blood. In essence, ultraviolet blood irradiation, or UBI, energizes the blood. It also aids in building up red blood cell count and eliminating toxins in the liver.

Like the other oxygenation therapies I've already covered, photoluminescence provokes an *indirect* attack on pathogenic microorganisms by triggering a chemical reaction inside cell membranes, which improves their ability to naturally fight infections. Blood cells also capture solar energy and use it to "radiate" cancer cells—almost like a natural form of radiation treatment that you'd receive from an oncologist only without harming your healthy cells! The Colorado Integrative Medical Center explains exactly how it works:

> Ultraviolet Blood Irradiation, simply called UBI, is a simple, painless and safe means of treating a person for a variety of illnesses. The procedure involves removing about 200 cc of blood (about the amount in a typical glass of water) and passing the blood through a quartz cuvette where it is exposed to ultraviolet light and returned to the blood stream. The ultraviolet light used is the same wave length produced by sunlight.

I hope you're beginning to see, if you haven't come to this conclusion already, that our bodies are *amazingly equipped* to handle disease on their own when given the proper tools to do so—or rather, when the tools that God built into us for such purposes are well maintained and functioning as they should. When they're not, it takes an intervention like UBI to make things right.

If your damaged cellular system was a set of dull steak knives, UBI would be the sharpener that goes around honing each one. UBI and the other oxygenation therapies I've covered don't actually *supplant* the knives; they just help them do their job *better*. In the case of solar energy, the immune system literally soaks it right up and uses it to forge a stronger assault against cancer. It's an incredibly simple process when you really think about it, yet the complexity of how it works internally

THE TRUTH ABOUT CANCER

with all the various moving parts melding together in perfect harmony is profoundly complex. To me, it's an awe-inspiring reflection of the unmatched intelligence and beauty of our Creator, who fashioned our bodies with the capacity to self-heal in ways that modern medicine can't even come close to replicating.

WHAT YOU NEED TO KNOW

- Oxygen is essential to proper cellular function; without it, your cells turn anaerobic and disease flourishes.
- If you body is besieged in an anaerobically dominated state, you may require bio-oxidative therapy in the form of ozone, hydrogen peroxide, intravenous vitamin C, or ultraviolet B (UVB) blood irradiation therapy.

CHAPTER 12

TREATING CANCER WITH VIRUSES AND ESSENTIAL OILS

When it comes to bacteria, there are both good kinds and bad kinds. The good kinds we typically consume in the form of fermented foods like those made from dairy (yogurt, cheese, cottage cheese, kefir), vegetables (kimchi, sauerkraut, pickles), and tea (kombucha), as well as naturally "probiotic" foods like spirulina, chlorella, and blue-green algae.[1] These "living" foods help keep our immune systems strong while protecting against bad bacteria like *Escherichia coli* (*E. coli*) and salmonellosis (*Salmonella*) that can make us very sick.

Probiotics are becoming all the rage these days because science is rapidly uncovering this missing piece in the health puzzle: much of what the average person eats on a daily basis is critically lacking in probiotic bacteria, which creates vulnerability to invasion by harmful pathogens. This is why it's so important to pay close attention to your probiotic intake, making sure you get enough through food and/or supplementation.

I'm a huge advocate of probiotics because I understand their necessity as part of an efficacious anticancer lifestyle. But during my travels, I also learned about beneficial *viruses*, which was an entirely new concept to me. You don't necessarily eat or supplement with them, but these viruses are being used in the emerging field of virotherapeutics to treat chronic illnesses like cancer, in a powerfully effective way.

The idea of "friendly" viruses first gained mainstream attention in 2013 when researchers from San Diego State University (SDSU) discovered a duality among viruses similar to that of bacteria. Certain viruses, they found, have the ability to complement the immune system and ward off disease by enhancing the protective ability of mucus membranes, which exist in the mouth, eyes, nose, and perhaps most importantly, the digestive tract.

SDSU microbiologist Jeremy Barr found that mucus is interlaced with both phages and viruses whose job it is to infect and destroy pathogenic microbes. Healthy mucus contains multiple layers of complex substances, including proteins, sugars, and what we now know to be disease-fighting viruses, or phages, that form a type of protective matrix around cells.

These seemingly unusual phages are what first caught the eye of Barr and his team, which decided to conduct tests on them to identify their purpose. They came to the realization that mucus contains "a soup of nutrients" that's fully equipped to deal with harmful microbes, and phages are a vital frontline in this multilayered defensive system.

"Mucus is actually a really cool and complex substance," Barr told *Science* magazine following the discovery. It's a novel immune system that we think is applicable to all mucosal surfaces, and it's one of the first examples of a direct symbiosis between phages and an animal host."[2]

In other words, viruses are an important part of a balanced immune ecosystem. Just as with bacteria, if they're not present or are present in improper amounts, symbiosis simply isn't possible.

GENETICALLY MODIFIED VIRUSES: IS THIS REALLY THE ANSWER?

In an attempt to capitalize on this groundbreaking discovery, drug manufacturers have been working on various virotherapies to use in the treatment of cancer. One, which was approved last fall by the FDA, is made from genetically engineered herpes virus, and it's said to provoke an immune response against cancer.[3] Member of a class of drugs known as "oncolytic" viruses, the transgenic viral treatment, called talimogene laherparepvec, or T-VEC, represents just one of more than a dozen oncolytic viruses currently undergoing clinical testing. The goal is to release a series of man-made viruses that Big Pharma can use to rake in the big bucks, now that many of their former blockbuster drugs are going off patent.

But do they work, and are they safe? Hardly. As I covered in one of my newsletters, T-VEC lacks the selective targeting ability that natural disease-fighting viruses have: it sweeps both healthy and unhealthy cells into the dustbin. And because it's made from the herpes virus, T-VEC can also lead to herpes viral infection. Its effectiveness is also questionable, as evidenced by the findings of a multicenter clinical trial submitted to the FDA. Only about 16.3 percent of patients treated with T-VEC, which is used to fight melanoma, experienced any sort of relief from their conditions. And if their melanomas had already gone metastatic, the drug's success was found to be *next to nil.*

RIGVIR: A NATURAL VIROTHERAPY FOR TREATING CANCER

I don't know about you, but this isn't the type of drug therapy I would *ever* consider using, especially when there are better options out there. One of these is RIGVIR, a *safe and effective* form of virotherapy that's becoming wildly popular in Europe. (It has yet to be accepted as a viable treatment here in the U.S.) Made from phages that exist naturally inside in the human body, RIGVIR belongs in a whole different class than genetically modified oncolytic drugs because it's both *oncotropic* and *oncolytic*: it selectively *targets* and *destroys* cancer cells. Healthy cells are unharmed by RIGVIR, which simply can't be said for FDA-approved oncolytic drugs.

The International Virotherapy Center in Riga, Latvia, is where RIGVIR was first developed, and it's also where the treatment is administered. People from all over the world travel there to gain access to this powerful therapy, which Dr. Kaspars Losans, M.D., former medical director of the center and one of its oncologists, says is incredibly effective. He told me that RIGVIR is the world's first clinically proven virotherapeutic medicine that's fully registered in Latvia as an accepted and viable treatment for cancer. It identifies and pursues cancer cells, making them visible to the immune system so they can be destroyed. This is one of the jobs of phages—to draw cancer cells out of hiding and into view. "[Cancer cells] have a natural ability to [hide] from the immune system," he explained to me. "Due to RIGVIR's guidance, because RIGVIR is attached, the viruses is attached to cancer, and RIGVIR [goes] inside the cancer cell. So the immune system, due to RIGVIR, recognizes cancer and starts to react against this cancer."

Though it's unclear how, or even whether or not, RIGVIR goes after cancer *stem* cells, Dr. Losans showed me compelling evidence to suggest that it does, very effectively. Many a successful patient has come out of the center with a clean bill of health thanks to RIGVIR treatment, many of them in a last-ditch effort after conventional therapies failed them. Even folks with late-stage cancers that the system ruled "incurable" have found true healing with RIGVIR, which serves as an amazing testimony to its efficacy.

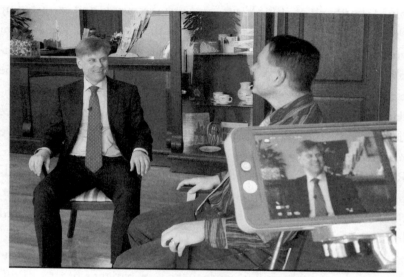

With Dr. Kaspars Losans in Riga, Latvia

"We have the largest experience yet accumulated for virotherapy with RIGVIR, so patients today come from more than 40 countries . . . to get this treatment and to be cured from their cancers."

Named after the city in which it was founded, RIGVIR, a combined shorthand of "Riga Virus," was first discovered and extracted by Professor Aina Muceniece. Familiar with the pre–World War I use of viruses as a treatment for cancer—the rabies vaccine being one example—Muceniece got to work trying to find others that might do the same thing. After isolating and testing a number of potential candidates from the stomachs and intestines of young children, Muceniece decided on RIGVIR because it is both *stable* and *nonmutating*, two requirements for a virus to be considered therapeutic. On top of that, RIGVIR is selectively toxic, demonstrating effectiveness in the treatment of cancers of the skin, kidneys, gastrointestinal tract, lungs, breast, prostate, and uterus, among others (though it's currently only approved for use in treating melanoma).

"Unlike the chemotherapy and the radiation therapy, this medicine does not leave such serious consequences in patient's organs," Prof. Muceniece once stated, and the rest is history.[4]

Again, just to reiterate, the GMO virotherapies gaining approval here in the U.S. aren't selective, nor are they nonmutating, which is why T-VEC can potentially lead to herpes infection in some patients. Such viruses are unpredictable and questionably beneficial at best; at worst, they're more harmful than they are beneficial, and not even worth using.

RIGVIR IS NOT A VACCINE

Not to be confused with a typical inoculation, RIGVIR, despite being an injection, is *not* a vaccine. Dr. Ivars Kalvins, an inventor, scientist, and partner at the center, explained to me what differentiates RIGVIR from a vaccine: "A normal vaccine is used to activate the immune system against the protein applied. . . . But RIGVIR [does not] invoke this immune response. It is going to find, or search for, cancer cells to penetrate into these cells. And then it will replicate inside of the cells by using all the factory mechanisms of these cells."

Because there are no foreign proteins involved in triggering an artificial immune response as there is with vaccines, there is little to no risk of complications from RIGVIR because the immune system isn't being unnaturally provoked and told to attack something that might cause an allergic reaction or worse, organ damage.

This is what sets RIGVIR apart from the rest, and it's one of the reasons why it's become so popular throughout the world. It's a one-of-a-kind treatment with a truly incredible track record of success, which is why people are willing to travel hundreds or even thousands of miles to Latvia to receive it.

VIROTHERAPY PROVOKES HYPERTHERMIC REACTION

Before I share with you some of the success stories that have emerged from the International Virotherapy Center, I'd like to explain another little tidbit about RIGVIR that I find fascinating in light of what we covered in the last chapter. Since RIGVIR contains a live virus, it often provokes a hyperthermic response in the body; basically, it causes a slight increase in temperature.

Many people see this as a "side effect" of the injection, but in this case it's actually a normal response to the body's immune system encountering the virus. As the virus draws cancer cells out of their hiding places, a "warming" effect occurs that not only gets the eradication process going, but also fires up the immune system. "The one side effect, the potential low-grade fever, is actually a good effect because it shows that your immune system is responding to the virus," says Dr. Losans.

Once again, we see the power of heat energy combined with natural organisms assisting the body in wiping out disease and restoring health. When a compromised immune system is fortified to do the job it was designed to do, disease simply doesn't stand a chance: the cure is your *immune system,* in other words, and heat, beneficial organisms, nutrients, and other supporting factors are merely the armament in this fight.

TESTIMONIES OF SUCCESSFUL RIGVIR TREATMENT

I got the chance to speak with a number of people who were treated with RIGVIR for various cancers, and I have to tell you that their stories really touched me, as I'm sure they will you. Many of these people were at the brink of losing all hope before trying RIGVIR, and now they've been healed and are living vibrant lives free of cancer.

A woman from Ukraine named Khrystyna Yakonvenko overcame stage IV melanoma after being treated with RIGVIR at the International Virotherapy Center. When this late-stage cancer spread to her liver, Khrystyna decided to take the advice of her conventional doctors back home and try palliative chemotherapy, which didn't work. She was told she would only live another six months. But Khrystyna decided to give RIGVIR a try because she figured, what could it hurt? She had already tried everything else and was basically being pronounced preliminarily *dead*, so why not see what happens? It would be the best decision she ever made, and one that I hope will inspire you and your loved ones, should you ever experience a cancer diagnosis.

"When I first came to the RIGVIR therapy center, the doctors didn't say that, yes, we will do it—they said, we will try, because the stage is late," Khrystyna told me as tears came streaming down her face. "I think that sometimes [during] the earlier stages . . . people who have this

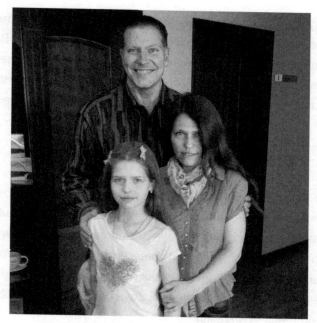

With Khrystyna and her daughter in Riga

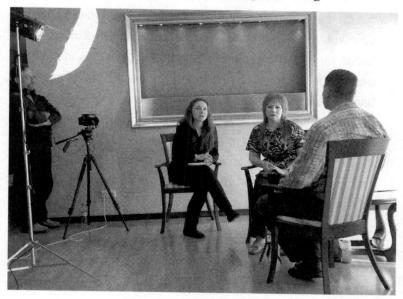

With Zoya in Riga

very scary diagnosis, they sometimes by themselves, they lose hope, they stop fighting, and they simply leave it. But sometimes there are people who, even at the late stages, they continue to fight, they continue to find the way out of the situation, and in this case, the disease is simply just over."

Khrystyna belongs to the latter group.

So does Zoya Sokolova of Russia, though her diagnosis was stage III sarcoma. Like Khrystyna and many others who make hasty decisions out of fear and coercion, Zoya went the conventional treatment route and almost died before stumbling upon RIGVIR. A major surgery followed by multiple rounds of chemotherapy left Zoya bedridden and unable to do much of anything.

Seeing her in the throes of passing, Zoya's family went out on a limb on her behalf, loading her up into the family's van and trekking several hundred miles across Europe to Latvia for RIGVIR treatment. Mind you, Zoya was in such bad shape just prior to arriving at the center that doctors back in Russia said her blood composition was *worse* than that of a dead person. "The doctor said exactly, 'I'm not asking how you got here, I'm asking how are you still alive with this blood test?'" she explained to me. "From my feelings at that moment, I realized that I would not survive, and I felt how my body is failing from day to day."

Zoya had to do a few things to boost her immune system prior to taking RIGVIR because she was *that* ill. But it was ultimately worth it because after just two weeks of getting the treatment, Zoya was able to get up out of bed and walk. It was like a miracle, she recalled with tears of joy, and one that she wishes everyone could experience. "When I started to receive RIGVIR therapy, very quickly I became a very healthy person. I started to travel, I started to have a lot of energy and I called [my friends] and I recommended that they start this treatment."

Zoya, of course, was familiar with other women like her back in Russia who were suffering from similar cancer diagnoses because she had met them while undergoing chemotherapy. I wish I could say that all of them took Zoya's advice after seeing her amazing recovery, but sadly most of them didn't. "It's a pity that a lot of great people are gone now," she lamented. "But I'm happy, I'm healthy, and I can't say that at the beginning I didn't trust this method, simply I didn't know and I was so weak. But now, currently, I don't have any more disabilities, I'm a completely healthy person and I'm so thankful to the people who have helped me here."

Hearing these kinds of stories brings such joy to my heart. To see people who thought they had one foot in the grave make full recoveries after just a few months of safe, noninvasive, nontoxic therapy speaks volumes to the power of progressive cancer treatments like RIGVIR.

I spoke to many other people who've been treated with RIGVIR and they all have similar testimonies:

- Karlis Venskus, who was cured of stage IV stomach cancer
- Egidijus Kazlauskis, who was cured of stage II melanoma
- Gunars Strazdinsh, who was cured of stage III small cell lung cancer
- Ruslan Isayev, who was cured of stage II skin melanoma
- Svetlana Sheferova, who was cured of stage III melanoma

Despite RIGVIR's incredible effectiveness, the treatment is currently *not* available in the U.S. because it's not a multimillion-dollar "block-buster" drug that can make drug companies rich. The only virus-related therapies legally offered are the ones I mentioned earlier: the genetically modified, therapeutically stunted, and highly unpredictable types offered at a premium by Big Pharma.

Having to travel across an ocean just to receive a real treatment that's *safe* and that *works* is unacceptable in a country that claims to be founded upon liberty and justice for all. But as the truth about cancer continues to proliferate, my hope is that things will eventually change—and hopefully *sooner* rather than later!

WHAT ABOUT ESSENTIAL OILS?

There's another way to improve the inner workings of your immune system, and it involves tapping into the immune systems of *plants*. You've probably never thought of plants as even having immune systems, but they do, and we call these *essential oils*: the botanical extracts of plant leaves that possess an array of protective chemical compounds.

Plants are just as susceptible to pestilence and disease as humans, and the way they protect themselves from the threat of viruses, fungi, bacteria, insects, and other invaders is with the fragrant, antioxidant-dense organic compounds they produce in their leaves and stems, compounds that when extracted can provide the same benefits for humans.

According to the National Association for Holistic Aromatherapy, plants use the essential oils they make:

- To attract pollinators and dispersal agents
- To deter the nearby growth of competing plants, a process known as allelopathy

- To defend against insects and other animals

- To protect against fungi and bacteria[5]

These same essential oils, which contain two classes of chemical constituents—hydrocarbons (mainly terpenes) and oxygenated compounds—have similar applicable uses in humans. I had the opportunity to speak with Dr. Eric Zielinski, D.C., a health coach and researcher with extensive knowledge in the use of essential oils as medicine, and what he told me was truly eye-opening.

I've long been familiar with the use of essential oils, particularly in aromatherapy, but like many people I had no idea that they could be used medicinally as a way to treat cancer. Despite their incredible diversity, essential oils seem to have one thing in common: virtually *all* of them possess anticancer properties.

In some parts of the world citrus is particularly abundant, so cultures there use the essential oils of citrus fruit to prevent and treat cancer. In other areas it's peppermint. And in still other areas it's melaleuca, tea tree, and eucalyptus. No matter where you go in the world, there seems to be some native plant life with an essential oil composition that's conducive to fighting cancer.

This is because essential oils in general contain compounds that stop angiogenesis, or the growth of veins and arteries, in cancer tumors. This means that essential oils are largely *antimetastatic*, as well as DNA protective, in many cases. Each one approaches cancer just slightly differently from the next, but they all play an important role in getting the job done of eradicating it—a joint effort known as *synergistic healing*. Dr. Zielinski explained:

> There is a research study that actually uses the terminology "synergistic approach." So in a sense, it's like this: Iron Man, he can kick butt. He's unstoppable. And the same thing with Captain America. But when you get them together, they save the world.

And that's exactly what research has found was in the chemicals in the essential oils. They work together in a synergistic approach, meaning this—you could take a ketone, you could take an ester out of an essential oil, and test that viability to kill certain cancer lines. But when you use the actual essential oil itself, it is a synergistic approach. But when you combine other oils too, it's like, boom, Avengers Part Two.

ORAL, TOPICAL, AND AROMATHERAPY

There are three ways to take essential oils: orally, topically, and diffused in the air as aromatherapy. Believe it or not, aromatherapy seems to be the most effective way to benefit from essential oils simply because the nerve endings in our nasal mucosa pick up the various organic compounds upon contact and immediately send them into the brain, where the hypothalamus begins utilizing them for therapeutic function. Both topical and oral intake of essential oils have their place in medicine, but these delivery methods don't work nearly as quickly as breathing in these organic compounds for instant effect.

"Not to use a crude analogy, but it's the best one that I have come up with," Dr. Zielinski told me, casually. "The reason why cocaine addicts snort cocaine instead of injecting cocaine is it's the fastest way of getting high . . . that is the most important way, in my opinion, to get the whole body affecting in a positive way."

Nutrition expert and author Dr. Josh Axe, D.N.M., D.C., C.N.S., of DrAxe.com has firsthand experience with essential oils. His mother successfully used oil of oregano as part of a natural treatment regimen for stage IV cancer, and along with juicing daily and supplementing with probiotics, she's now living a healthy, vibrant life. "One of the things that she had chronic issues with is digestive issues," Dr. Axe told me. "She had leaky gut, chronic constipation, and severe issues with yeast. So she was constantly craving sugar. She even developed a toenail fungus, major yeast and candida issues. Oil of oregano is packed with

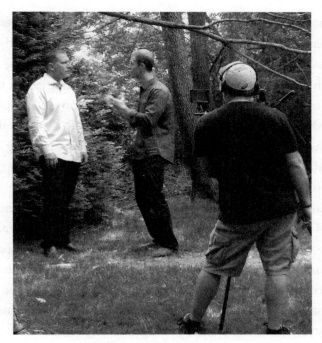

With Dr Josh Axe in Nashville

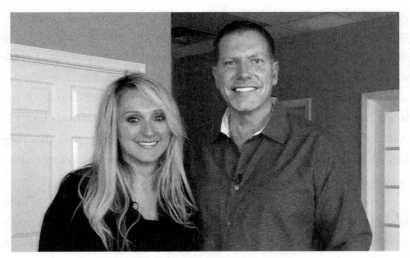

With Allison Huish in Atlanta

some incredible compounds, thymol, carvacrol . . . we started doing [it], three drops, three times a day internally, as well as topically on the toenail . . . and after two months it completely cleared up the issue."

Even more powerful than oil of oregano for treating cancer is frankincense oil, which Dr. Axe says is one of the most powerful supplements *period* when it comes to destroying cancer cells. Rich in a substance known as boswellia, or boswellic acid, frankincense is a strong anti-inflammatory and antioxidant oil that studies have shown has an amazing ability to shrink cancer tumors.

There have been about seven studies published on the anticancer effects of frankincense oil, though nearly all of them are *in vitro*, meaning they were conducted in petri dishes rather than in living animals or humans. One *in vivo* study looking at the a-Pinene chemotype in frankincense oil showed efficacy in the treatment of pancreatic cancer, while many other *in vitro* studies showed benefits to this and other compounds in treating bladder, breast, colorectal, skin, and other forms of cancer.

One particular cancer for which frankincense oil shows incredible promise as a treatment is cancer of the brain. Its molecular size is so small that it can easily pass into brain tissue and take on any lingering inflammation, jump-starting the immune response in pursuit of eradicating cancer cells. "Most everybody knows that in cancer treatment, chemotherapy is not effective at treating any sort of cancer of the brain because it can't pass through the blood-brain barrier," says Dr. Axe. "Versus frankincense oil, those compounds are so small that they can actually pass through the blood-brain barrier and start to reduce neural inflammation."

One woman who approached Dr. Axe following one of his talks told him about how frankincense oil cured her husband's supposedly terminal brain cancer. He was told he only had three months to live, but after taking frankincense oil daily, both vaporized and applied to the roof of his mouth, he proved his doctors wrong. "We diffused it in the home, we rubbed it on the roof of his mouth. It's been six years and he's still alive and we really believe it's because of this use of frankincense oil."

To get even more of the active ingredient boswellia, some experts recommend using frankincense *extract* rather than the oil. The Tisserand Institute says even a high-quality frankincense extract only has about 1 percent boswellic acid, while a well-suited extract contain anywhere between 40 and 60 percent boswellic acid.[6]

If you recall the story of the three magi, or wise men, from the Bible who traveled from the East to see the newborn Christ, you might remember that they brought with them gold, frankincense, and myrrh as gifts. The latter two weren't just meant to be used as fragrance, but also as medicine. Much like frankincense, myrrh performs a series of functions in the body that make it, too, a useful remedy in treating cancer. Myrrh is powerful, says Dr. Axe, because it works directly on the hypothalamus and the liver to reduce inflammation. It's also a hormone balancer, which is critical for fighting estrogen-based cancers like those of the breast.

If people have heard of indole-3-carbinol or the benefits of cruciferous vegetables—it works in a very similar manner, but in a more potent way to where it really helps clear the body of excess estrogen or xenoestrogens that are found in things like soy and plastics and parabens today. It also really helps detoxify the liver and also boost a very important antioxidant called glutahione, which supports detoxification.

So if you really think about it, taking both frankincense *and* myrrh together can tackle cancer from two different angles. A study published in the journal *Oncology Letters* in 2013 looked at how the essential oils of frankincense and myrrh affected five different tumor cells lines, determining that while the two substances aren't necessarily *synergistic*, per se, they both exhibit anticancer effects.[7]

And there are all sorts of other essential oils with their own anticancer properties as well, including:

- Lavender
- Sandalwood
- Lemongrass
- Wintergreen
- Fir needle
- Lemon
- Lime

And the list goes on and on, with literally *hundreds* of essential oil varieties showing efficacy in the cancer treatment department. Similar to cannabis, which comes in a wide variety of strains, each with its own unique therapeutic profile, the plants from which essential oils are extracted also contain their own distinctive array of terpenes, terpenoids, phenolic (aromatic) components, and aliphatic (alkanes and alkenes) compounds that render them uniquely therapeutic, and yet mutually beneficial.

"Most of EOs have been first identified and used for the treatment of inflammatory and oxidative diseases," reads a systematic review of more than 100 essential oils from 20 different plant families that was published in the *American Journal of Cancer Research*. "It appeared that these EOs could also have anticancer effects as there is a relationship between the production of reactive oxygen species to the origin of oxidation and inflammation that can lead to cancer. . . . Chronic inflammation has been linked to various steps involved in carcinogenesis, such as cellular transformation, promotion, survival, proliferation, invasion, angiogenesis, and metastasis. Several studies have thus shown that EOs and their components therein could be active against various cancer cells."[8]

I got a chance to speak to a woman named Allison Huish who used essential oils to overcome a brain stem tumor that she was diagnosed with at the age of 13. It was a pilocytic astrocytoma, a type of tumor that is typically only found in six- or seven-year-old boys, *not* teenage girls. Her chiropractor believed that this rare and unusual tumor was the result of Allison having been vaccinated for DPT (diphtheria, pertussis, and tetanus), but whatever the case, she still had to deal with it.

Allison's family knew about the antitumor effects of frankincense oil, as well as its ability to boost white blood cell count (white blood cells, remember, help fight off disease). She combined the use of this oil with oil of clove and other plants while also cleaning up her diet, and almost immediately her brain tumor began to shrink. Within about three years, she was confirmed to be completely tumor free.

"I don't care what the diagnosis is. I don't care what the number is. Don't believe it," essential oil expert Dr. Zielinksi, also a friend of Allison's, passionately expressed to me during an interview. "Believe that God's given you an unbelievable ability to heal yourself, as Allison found out."

WHAT YOU NEED TO KNOW

- "Good" bacteria help to keep the body oxygenated naturally while fending off "bad" bacteria that cause disease.

- Regular intake of probiotic foods and beverages helps to keep both gut and oral ecology in balance, minimizing the risk of disease.
- There are also "good" viruses that help protect the body against 'bad" viruses, and virotherapies like RIGVIR can help bolster the former when the latter take over and cause problems.
- Virotherapy also provokes a hyperthermic (heat) response in the body, further dealing with the factors of disease.
- Essential oils are selectively-toxic immune boosters that go after harmful pathogens—bacterial, viral, fungal, and otherwise—while protecting benign ones.

CHAPTER 13

ENZYME AND METABOLIC/ MITOCHONDRIAL THERAPY

When a large company decides to cut its costs by merging departments and offloading dead weight, perhaps bringing in a consultant to help expedite the job of "cleaning house," we call this process corporate restructuring. It happens all the time in the business world as a way to maximize efficiency and ensure that the highest-quality goods and services are made available to customers at the lowest possible prices.

It's a routine *survival* tactic that has many parallels with the way our bodies work. Particularly with regard to the cellular system, the human body is designed to target both malignant and dead cells that interfere with healthy ones so they can be flushed out of the body, improving the overall "quality of life" for healthy cells that as a result are able to function at optimal capacity—a win-win for the state of *your* health.

Previously we've talked about apoptosis, a process of programmed cell death by which the immune system takes care of cancer cells before they start to go rogue and form tumors, spreading metastatically. But there's another process of programmed cell *life* that we refer to as autophagy, which literally means "self-eating," that's absolutely critical for health maintenance and disease prevention.

Similar to a corporate restructuring consultant, autophagy is the body's way of scouring the cellular matrix for waste in order to dispose of and/or recycle it. The primary purpose of autophagy is to pick up the trash, so to speak, whether it be intracellular viruses, protein aggregates, bacteria, subcellular organelles, or damaged proteins, *and get rid of these by whatever means possible.*

Autophagy, in a nutshell, is a promoter of life rather than death. It acts as a type of "grease" in the gears of the natural cellular degradation process, and serves as a mechanism for continuous cellular maintenance and regeneration. It also streamlines the process of waste removal in the body, which, as you'll see, is a vital part of metabolic normalcy.

Autophagocytosis, another name for autophagy, is also relevant in the functionality of the neurological system. A study published in the journal *Experimental Neurobiology* explains how the neuronal system, the means by which cells communicate with one another, is intrinsically dependent upon autophagy for its growth and repair. "Neurons have highly dynamic cellular processes for their proper functions such as cell growth, synaptic formation, or synaptic plasticity by regulating protein synthesis and degradation," the study reveals, noting that "the quality control of proteins in neurons is essential for their physiology and pathology."[1]

Autophagy, by its very nature, operates within the realm of cellular digestion and enzyme production, and this is why researchers are increasingly pointing to its dysfunction as a factor in neurological disease. It also protects the communication apparatus of cells, a breakdown of which can lead to brain diseases like Alzheimer's and dementia, not to mention cancer. If neuronal pathways aren't constantly being cleared of waste buildup, they eventually lose their ability to function at all. This is why autophagocytosis is so important.

Many experts now surmise that autophagy is the single greatest factor in the aging process, in fact, as evidenced by the fact that *when it's functioning as it should,* free radical damage and cellular dysfunction are virtually nonexistent, or at least kept to a *minimum.* "There is much stronger evidence of a link between autophagy activation and longevity than there is with any other longevity interventions such as exogenous antioxidant supplementation, endogenous antioxidant up-regulation, micronutrient replacement, hormone replacement, anti-inflammatory therapy, telomerase activation, or stem cell therapy," writes Dr. James P. Watson, M.D., an expert in the molecular biology of aging.[2]

Just to reiterate, autophagy is the catabolic process by which cells constantly degrade their own unneeded cell components in order to promote new cell growth and maintain homeostasis. It's the mechanism through which balance is achieved between the synthesis, degradation, and recycling of cellular components, all for the purpose of optimizing cellular function. Autophagy lies at the heart of cancer prevention and it's how our bodies attain *and maintain* optimal health.

Understanding how this process works gives relevance to the cellular life cycle and turns popular cancer theory on its head. While the cancer system remains fixated on gene mutations as the root cause of cancer and unleashes failed drug treatment after failed drug treatment targeted toward them, the reality is that DNA damage is merely a *symptom* of autophagic breakdown, which can only be addressed with therapies that restore metabolic normalcy.

It's what Otto Warburg hypothesized in 1924 about the true nature of cancer. He proposed, facing much opposition from his peers, that cancer isn't a genetic disease but rather a *metabolic* disease characterized by damaged cellular metabolism. Mitochondrial dysfunction, in other words—*not* genetic predisposition—is why otherwise healthy cells suddenly switch to an anaerobic state and become cancerous. This is the very foundation of the metabolic theory of cancer, which posits that genetic mutations are secondary symptoms of cancer. Science affirms this, yet the cancer industry has shown little concern with trying to set the record straight and has, in fact, gone to great lengths to *suppress* this vital truth from gaining traction in the public consciousness.[3]

Boston University professor Thomas Seyfried describes cancer as a metabolic disease that alters the "entire complexion of the cell." And genetic mutations, he says, are just one damaging by-product among many that exacerbate this systemic destabilization process, which lies at the root of *most* (but not all) cancers.[4]

Comprehensive DNA sequencing has shown that the mutation signatures of individual cancers vary dramatically from tumor to tumor, and even from cell to cell within the same tumor. This renders the targeted drug model futile, as trying to tackle cancer by focusing on eradicating DNA mutations is like shooting at a moving target—or as Dr. Ira Goodman, M.D., puts it, "a multibillion-dollar wild goose chase after the wrong target."[5]

As for metastasis, the death sentence of nearly every cancer diagnosis, DNA sequencing as a treatment approach has likewise proven to be a spectacular failure for the very same reasons.

"Comprehensive sequencing was unable to find a single mutation responsible for the most important quality of cancer, the single feature of cancer responsible for 90% of all cancer deaths," writes Travis Christofferson in his book *Tripping Over the Truth*, which outlines experiments demonstrating the fruitlessness of going after nuclear DNA in an attempt to eradicate cancer.[6]

So if damaged DNA isn't responsible for initiating metabolic disease, what is? Like any other bodily system, cellular metabolism can be brought into disarray due to a number of factors, not the least of which include nutrient deficiencies, toxic overload, and chronic stress. Insufficient enzyme intake, which I touched on earlier, is also implicated in autophagic breakdown, hence the growing use of enzyme therapy as a way to bring it back up to speed.

ENZYME THERAPY AND CANCER

The late Dr. Nicholas Gonzalez, M.D., advocated for the use of pro-teolytic enzyme therapy as a treatment for cancer because, based on the findings of a number of case studies, it's an unquestionably effective way to optimize autophagocytosis. The idea originally came from embryologist Dr. John Beard, who in 1906 made the proposition that proteolytic digestive enzymes are effective in the treatment of *all* types of cancer due to their being the body's *primary* defense against cancer.

After his death in 1923, Dr. Beard's ideas and methods fell into obscurity for a time, only to reemerge in the early 1980s. Dr. Gonzalez met Dr. William Donald Kelley, a dentist from Texas, who was using proteolytic enzymes to treat cancer patients. Dr. Gonzalez later adopted the therapy as part of his individualized nutrition protocols for cancer, which, despite his recent and unfortunate death, are still being used at his New York clinic.

A monograph put together by Dr. Gonzalez back in 1986 as part of his fellowship training program in medical school reveals how enzyme therapy has helped many cancer patients who were told they had only months or even *weeks* to live go on to survive for *years*: a formidable *cure* for cancer, if you ask me. After bringing the treatment back to his clinic, Dr. Gonzalez saw firsthand the positive effects of enzyme therapy in his patients, the evidence of which he presented before the National Cancer Institute's associate director for the Cancer Therapy Evaluation Program, Dr. Linda Isaacs. This evidence was so compelling to Dr. Isaacs that she proposed conducting a pilot study on the treatment in patients with one of the most incurable forms of cancer:

cancer of the pancreas. The results of the study were published in the journal *Nutrition and Cancer* in 1999, revealing the following:

> Of 11 patients followed in the trial, 8 of 11 suffered stage IV disease. Nine of 11 (81 percent) lived one year, 5 of 11 lived two years (45 percent), 4 of 11 lived three years (36 percent) and two lived longer than four years. In comparison, in a trial of the drug gemcitabine, of 126 patients with pancreatic cancer not a single patient lived longer than 19 months.[7]

The NCI and the National Center for Alternative and Complementary Medicine would go on to fund a large-scale trial not long after that. But because of mismanagement by the academicians involved—these scientists, according to Dr. Gonzalez, failed to ensure that patients were following the strict nutritional guidelines set forth for the study—it didn't come to the same conclusions. A follow-up investigation conducted by the Office of Human Research Protections, an investigative arm of the National Institutes of Health, verified that researchers at Columbia University had mismanaged the study, a fact that was also affirmed by the FDA. But that didn't stop Dr. Gonzalez and his team from making sure truth won out.

A peer-reviewed study published in the journal *Pancreas* in 2004,[8] which was included as part of a lengthy review published in the journal *Alternative Therapies in Health and Medicine* in 2007,[9] show that proteolytic enzyme therapy is indeed an effective treatment against pancreatic and many other forms of cancer. Dr. Gonzalez's clinic utilizes it alongside a rigorous diet and detoxification protocol for maximum benefits. "The therapy itself is quite complex, but basically involves three components: diet, aggressive supplementation with nutrients and pancreas product (containing naturally occurring enzymes), and detoxification," the clinic says. "The protocols are individualized and each patient receives a diet designed for his or her specific needs. The diets are quite variable, ranging from a pure vegetarian program to a diet requiring fatty red meat 2–3 times a day."

For a person who already has cancer, the required daily dosage of pancreatic enzyme supplements is rather intense; it can range from anywhere between 130 and 175 capsules per *day*. These supplements contain a range of trace elements, minerals, vitamins, antioxidants, and animal glandular products, again customized for each patient's particular needs.

The most important part of the protocol is the pancreatic product, which is derived from animals raised in the pristine environments of Australia and New Zealand, where the animal husbandry standards are the highest in the world. And this is accompanied by an aggressive detoxification regimen that helps rid the body of all the metabolic waste products and stored toxins that are released during the therapy's highly effective "repair and rebuild" phase.[10]

The story behind how Dr. Gonzalez came to practice this type of functional medicine is an incredible one, especially because he was trained conventionally at Cornell University. It was a matter of being in the right place at the right time, and being open minded enough to take a somewhat divergent path than his peers, that made Dr. Gonzalez a legend in the cancer treatment world. His nutritional training under Dr. Kelley combined with his mentorship under former Memorial Sloan Kettering Cancer Center president Robert Good allowed Dr. Gonzalez to rise in the ranks very quickly and become a leader in the proper application of enzyme- and nutritional-based therapies for treating cancer. Dr. Gonzalez's individualized approach to patient care was birthed out of his training under Dr. Kelley, who came up with 10 different diets, as well as 94 variations of these diets, that he "prescribed" to his patients. Because every individual has a unique biological and physiological makeup, he realized, no one dietary approach would work for everyone as some kind of one-size-fits-all cure.

But it's the enzymes that really do the work. As Dr. Gonzalez explained to me, they seem to selectively target the proteins on cancer cell membranes and "chew them up," as he put it, though the precise mechanism of action has yet to be fully fleshed out due to a lack of rigorous testing. "Cell membranes are a little bit fatty but they also have protein molecules that are receptors, and pores that allow nutrients to get in, and waste products to get out . . . that is how cells survive, with the protein pores and membrane. These proteins—I think the enzymes chew them up. They don't affect normal tissue," he told me, with the caveat, "but we haven't had the trillions of dollars of funding to substantiate that."

What we do have, though, are plenty of peer-reviewed clinical and animal models to show that the therapy works, not only at Dr. Gonzalez's clinic but also at that of Dr. Kelley, who successfully administered the treatment to his patients for many years. And Dr. Gonzalez credits not himself but his predecessors who came up with this comprehensive healing approach, which deals not only with cancer cells and tumors, but also tumor *waste* that so often causes patients to become ill—hence his focus on detoxification.

"They work for any type of cancer," Dr. Gonzalez told me about his enzymes. "That is why . . . I deliberately chose 26 different types of cancer (in my research)—50 patients and 26 different types of cancer—to make the point that it works for all different types of cancer. Leukemias, lymphomas, blood cancer, solid tumors, breast, colon, rectal, metastatic prostate, and a whole series of them."

But perhaps the most impressive of all is its effectiveness against pancreatic cancer, which is largely considered to be incurable. One of Dr. Kelley's patients, a woman named Arlene Van Straten from Appleton, Wisconsin, was cured of pancreatic cancer more than 30 years ago thanks to the enzyme therapeutic protocol still in use at Dr.

Gonzalez's clinic in New York City, a testament to its amazing potential as a universal cancer killer.

Another of Dr. Gonzalez's patients, Brenda Michaels, a 30-year breast cancer and cervical cancer survivor, shares her story:

I learned that I was extremely toxic, and that I needed to be detoxified. . . . I learned about coffee enemas, something that most people go, "Oh my God, don't tell me, don't share that with me." But when I learned about what the coffee bean holds and how it helps to open up those pores in the liver, to draw the toxins out of the liver, it made sense to me. So instead of pushing all that away, because for a lot of people the diet is so strict having to take the pills every so often and waking up in the middle of the night and having to do coffee enemas. Enzymes, vitamins, minerals. I was taking 143 different vitamins, minerals, and enzymes a day. Five days on, two days off. And then, in between, I was doing these very heavy detoxifying procedures that he has his patients do. . . . I'm in my 60s, I'm the healthiest I feel I've ever been.

METABOLIC THERAPY: GETTING RID OF CANCER-CAUSING WASTE

As you can see, Dr. Gonzalez's therapeutic approach is multipronged, encompassing diet, enzymes, and detoxification. Each piece is ultimately meant to get rid of the toxins in the body that weaken immunity

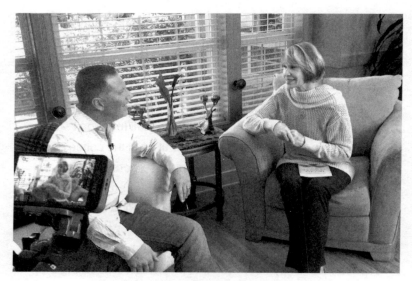

With Brenda Michaels in Seattle

and allow cancer to form, a comprehensive treatment philosophy that falls underneath the larger banner of *metabolic therapy*.

There are many types of metabolic therapy with a solid track record of success besides that of Dr. Gonzalez and his predecessor Dr. Kelley, including the famous Gerson Therapy, Issels Immunotherapy, the macrobiotic diet, the Contreras Metabolic Therapy, and various others. Some of these overlap in certain areas—several promote coffee enemas for bowel cleansing along with the removal of mercury dental fillings to eliminate heavy metal toxicity, and their general philosophies are largely the same—to strengthen the body's ability to ward off disease.

One common theme among virtually all forms of metabolic therapy is their focus on eating a *clean, whole food-based diet*, supplemented with vitamins and minerals. In the case of Gerson Therapy, the idea is to flood the body with the nutrients of between 15 and 20 pounds of organically grown fruits and vegetables *every single day*. Much of this is consumed as fresh juice, which is taken by the glass up to 13 times daily, once every hour.

The result? Improved oxygenation of blood and comprehensive elimination of toxins. The Gerson Institute explains:

> Oxygenation is usually more than doubled, as oxygen deficiency in the blood contributes to many degenerative disease. The metabolism is also stimulated through the addition of thyroid, potassium and other supplements, and by avoiding heavy animal fats, excess protein, sodium, and other toxins.
>
> Degenerative diseases render the body increasingly unable to excrete waste materials adequately, commonly resulting in liver and kidney failure. The Gerson Therapy uses intensive detoxification to eliminate wastes, regenerate the liver, reactivate the immune system and restore the body's essential defenses—enzyme, mineral and hormone systems. With generous, high-quality nutrition, increased oxygen availability, detoxification, and improved

metabolism, the cells—and the body—can regenerate, become healthy and prevent future illness.[11]

The Gerson Therapy is heavily centered around vegetables and other plant-based foods, as well as rigorous supplementation. Dr. Max Gerson was also a huge proponent of coffee enemas, which he believed help round out the therapy and maximize the elimination of cancer-fueling toxins.

Issels Immunotherapy takes a somewhat different approach, utilizing both specific and nonspecific therapies to target and eliminate cancer cells while creating "microenvironments" that are unfavorable to tumor growth and spread. The protocol involves the use of non-toxic vaccines, cell therapies, and personalized immunobiologic core treatments that are constantly being refined to work better and more quickly than previous iterations.

The Issels Clinic utilizes a combination of nutritional immuno-therapy, autohemotherapy (the same technique used in ozone therapy), enzymatic therapy, oxidative therapy, photoluminescence (ultraviolet light) therapy, laetrile therapy, polarizing solutions, glandular supple-mentation, phytotherapy, homeopathy, intravenous nutrition, nutra-ceuticals, psychological guidance, and physical therapy.

The three main components of Issels Immunotherapy include:[12]

Cancer-fighting vaccines
These vaccines provoke dendritic cells, the most potent among the antigen-forming cells in the body, to support both innate and adaptive immunity, while also stimulating the production of disease-fighting factors like interferons, interleukins, colony stimulating factors, and tumor necrosis factor.

Immune-enhancing protocols
Activated natural killer (NK) and lymphokine-activated killer (LAK) cells are introduced to destroy cancer cells while autologous cytokines are brought in to boost immunity. Stem cells help repair damaged

tissue and organs, while extracorporeal photopheresis provides immu-
nomodulatory benefits. And systemic hyperthermia, or full-body heating, is utilized to further promote immune function.

Comprehensive immunobiologic core treatment
This individually customized blend of nontoxic therapies helps destroy
cancer tumors while addressing the underlying immune deficiencies
that led to their formation. The purpose of this component is to rebuild
and activate the body's natural defenses against disease.

The macrobiotic diet was developed by Japanese philosopher George
Ohsawa in the 1920s as a way to try to improve humanity's coexistence
with nature. Ohsawa's belief was that consumption of *living, toxin-free*
foods is the best way to avoid *and cure* chronic disease—sound familiar?
That's because the macrobiotic philosophy complements enzyme therapy and many of the other alternative anticancer protocols I've outlined
in this book. Though typically customized for each individual, a true
macrobiotic diet is generally composed of the following:

- Organic whole grains—brown rice, barley, oats, and buck-
  wheat—as *half* of one's food intake
- Locally grown, organic fruits and vegetables as *one-quarter*
  of one's food intake
- Soups made from vegetables, seaweed, chick peas, beans,
  lentils, and miso (fermented soy), up to *one-quarter* of
  one's food intake

Just to be clear, I'm not necessarily advocating for this precise regimen—many would contend that consuming large amounts of grains
is cancer *forming* rather than cancer *preventing*—but I do think it's
important to cover because, for some people, adhering to this diet has
helped them overcome cancer.[13]

The late Dr. Ernesto Contreras from the Oasis of Hope Hospital in Tijuana, Mexico, developed his own form of metabolic therapy that he dubbed the Contreras Alternative Cancer Treatment (C-ACT). Like Dr. Gonzalez's enzyme therapy, C-ACT is a multimodal therapeutic approach that's customized for each patient.

Depending on a patient's condition, he or she will be enrolled into one of two C-ACT protocols: C-ACT-Q, a combined treatment that includes cytotoxic chemotherapy; or C-ACT-C, the same protocol except instead of chemotherapy, a patient receives high-dose vitamin C injections.

The therapeutic elements of C-ACT include:[14]

Cell redox regulation therapy
High-dose vitamin C combined with vitamin K is injected intravenously to produce lethal amounts of hydrogen peroxide in tumors, effectively killing them.

Oxidative stress preconditioning
Ozone autohemotherapy and UV blood irradiation are utilized to precondition healthy cells to protect themselves against the oxidative stress associated with treatment.

Immune stimulation therapy
Immunosupportive agents like probiotics, coffee, and the hormone melatonin are used to boost the immune system's cancer-fighting abilities.

Signal transduction therapy
Nutrients, phytochemicals, and drugs are used to gain control over the signaling pathways of cancer cells in order to better control and destroy them.

Cytotoxic therapy
Once all these factors are in place, low-dose chemotherapy or other cytotoxic agents are used to deliver the final blow to cancer cells and tumors.

Emotional and spiritual support
Undergoing any type of treatment for cancer is tough, which is why the Oasis of Hope offers emotional counseling and spiritual encouragement for patients.

There are so many factors at play with cancer that a customized approach to dealing with it is really the only logical solution. I like the multimodal philosophy embraced by Oasis of Hope, Dr. Gonzalez, and others because it leaves no stone unturned in the battle against cancer. We often use the term *integrative* to describe this approach because that's exactly what it does: it integrates the healing power of nutrients, immune factors, oxygen, cytotoxins, light, sound, heat, enzymes, and more to hit cancer from every angle.

It's not enough to just target cancer cells with destruction because, in many cases, they know how to outsmart this assault and set up shop elsewhere in the body, while in the process mutating and becoming much stronger the second time around. And carpet bombing the body with poison and radiation just destroys *everything*, including the immune factors that would take care of cancer on their own if they were simply strong enough and equipped to do so. That's why a comprehensive treatment program that focuses on fortifying the immune system and prepping healthy cells for war is a critical part of the cancer treatment equation, especially for late-stage cancers that have already metastasized.

PROTEOLYTIC ENZYMES FOR EVERYDAY CANCER PREVENTION

If we recognize that proper mitochondrial function is the basis upon which our cells produce ATP, or cellular energy, then it follows that taking the necessary steps to ensure optimal mitochondrial function is critical for cancer prevention. And I would contend that one of the best ways to do this, both from a nutrition and a detoxification perspective, is with supplemental proteolytic enzymes.

A recent paper published in the journal *Nature Reviews Molecular Cell Biology* spells out exactly why proteolytic enzymes are so important: without them, cellular mitochondria are unable to synthesize proteins, induce cell apoptosis, eliminate waste, and perform other necessary functions integral to life. When these functions are inhibited, the consequences can be devastating: think neurodegenerative disease, metabolic syndrome, and cancer.[15]

This is why I can't emphasize enough the importance of supplementing with systemic, proteolytic enzymes, which, besides cleaning up the blood and improving lymphatic function, help to:

- Control systemic inflammation throughout the body
- Repair and rebuild the cardiovascular system
- Improve blood flow
- Clean up and optimize the immune system
- Prevent and dissolve blood clots and arterial plaque
- Increase exercise capacity and recovery times
- Break down rogue proteins in the soft tissue and blood

Jon Barron covers a lot of his in his report *Enzymes Defined*, which highlights the fact that there are upwards of 70,000 unique enzymes inside the body that regulate every single function—and we're not just talking about *digestive* enzymes, but rather systemic, or *metabolic*, enzymes that manage the way the body functions. "Proteolytic is a catchall phrase for hydrolytic enzymes that specifically facilitate the chemical breakdown of proteins by severing the bonds between the amino acids that make up those proteins," Barron writes. "They are different from other enzymes in the body in that they are able to adapt to changing needs."[16]

When you understand that all pathogens, allergens, and rogue cells (cancer cells) have protein defense shields, you'll also very quickly see why proteolytic enzymes, which possess unique protein degradation properties, are so essential for maintenance and waste removal. Proteolytic enzymes are arguably *the* most important factor in cancer prevention at the systemic level.

A good quality proteolytic enzyme formula will contain the following enzymes at their various activity levels:

- Protease, 300,000 HUT (hemoglobin units, tyrosine basis)
- Fungal pancreatin, 1,200 USP (United States Pharmacopeia)
- Nattokinase, 540 FU (fibrinolytic units), which refers to its ability to break down the blood-clotting enzyme fibrin
- Seaprose S, 15,000 U (enzyme unit)
- Papain, 72 MCU (milk clotting units), a measurement of how quickly this enzyme digests milk protein (sometimes listed as PU, or papain units, which are equivalent to 0.1 MCU)
- Bromelain, 336 GDU (gelatin digesting units), a measurement of how fast this enzyme digests gelatin (1 MCU is about 0.67 GDU)
- Amylase, 3,000 SKB (named after its test creators Sandstedt, Kneen, and Blish), sometimes labeled as DU (brewing measurement), with SKB and DU matching up at a 1:1 equivalency.
- Lipase, 192 FIP (test methodology of the Fédération Internationale Pharmaceutique)

The benefits of proteolytic enzyme supplementation are well worth the investment, and taking them regularly can make all the difference in cancer prevention. Your body will use them to:

- Destroy harmful bacteria, viruses, molds, and fungi
- Quell damaging inflammation
- Purify your blood
- Clean out your lungs
- Maximize immunity
- Dissolve scar tissue
- Promote systemic detoxification
- Eliminate autoimmune conditions

The key is to combine proteolytic enzymes with a diet centered around *more* raw and living foods and *fewer* cooked and processed foods. And remember to *chew* your food thoroughly and drink plenty of water throughout the day, as detoxification comes to a grinding halt when you're dehydrated.

RESTRICTED KETOGENIC DIET

Also known as R-KD, a Restricted Ketogenic Diet centers around starving out cancer cells by depriving them of the various substances on which they feed, while also continuing to support healthy cells. This means that, for the most part, carbohydrates (and to a lesser degree proteins, depending on the cancer) have to go, and fats have to take their place—lots and lots of fat!

When carbohydrates are no longer available for cellular fuel production, the body starts metabolizing fat as an alternate fuel, converting it into a unique class of compounds known as ketones. Cancer cells have no use for ketones, but healthy cells are able to quickly adapt to start using them as food, a win-win situation for treating cancer.

Professor Seyfried has conducted extensive study on ketones and found them to be both antiangiogenic (meaning they cut off the energy delivery systems of tumors and deprive them of nutrients) and proapoptotic (helping facilitate the orderly deaths of cancer cells). The goal is to put as much metabolic stress on cancer cells as possible, weakening their support systems to such a high degree that swooping in and wiping them out with adjunct therapies becomes almost effortless.

R-KD isn't typically administered as a stand-alone treatment for cancer, but rather as a complementary addition that enhances the cancer-fighting effects of other treatments like hyperbaric oxygen therapy. Combining these nontoxic therapies exploits the overlapping metabolic deficiencies of cancer, helping significantly decrease blood glucose and tumor growth rate while increasing survival rates.[17]

INTERMITTENT FASTING

Many people do it for cultural and religious purposes, but fasting has a place in cancer treatment as well—and I'm not even talking about having to starve yourself for days at a time in order to see results. Simply adjusting the *times* at which you eat, a protocol known as *intermittent* fasting, can make all the difference in getting your metabolism back on track.

It's something they do down at the Hope4Cancer Clinic in Tijuana as an adjunct to the other treatments offered there. Dialing down the time frames in which patients eat from the typical morning, noon, and night routine, which can span upwards of 12 hours or even longer, to a much smaller 6- to 8-hour window during the middle of the day has helped many people conquer their cancers faster and with greater comfort throughout the process.

Intermittent fasting has been shown to help boost insulin sensitivity and reduce insulin resistance, while at the same time promoting normalized autophagy. Oscar Puig, a nutritionist at the Hope4Cancer Institute, is keen on the "Leangains" Method of intermittent fasting, which restricts eating times to between noon and 8 P.M. every day. This method is both effective and easy to follow because the daily schedule remains the same rather than changing.[18]

You wouldn't think that depriving a person's body of nutrition during certain hours of the day would have much effect on his cancer state, but it does. A 2009 study out of the University of Southern California found that cells respond to this period of being in "starvation mode" differently depending on whether they're healthy or malignant.

Healthy cells generally wait out this "lean period" by going into a type of hibernation mode, which protects them from damage. But cancer cells continue to grow because their genetic pathways are stuck in "on" mode, which makes them less resistant to stress and more prone to failure.

"The cell is, in fact, committing cellular suicide," stated Valter Longo, an associate professor of gerontology and biology at the University of Southern California, who for years has been studying the effects of intermittent fasting on cancer and how cancer cells respond to this nontoxic therapy. "What we're seeing is that the cancer cell tries to compensate for the lack of all these things missing in the blood after fasting. It may be trying to replace them, but it can't."[19]

The fact of the matter is that *every* type of cancer is treatable with metabolic therapy, whether it involves intermittent fasting, R-KD, enzyme therapy, or some combination of all of these. As Professor Seyfried puts it, all types of cancer have "the same, beautiful, metabolic target" painted on their backs, which means beating this dreadful disease is simply a matter of hitting it, and hitting it hard.[20]

WHAT YOU NEED TO KNOW

- The human body is designed to efficiently remove dead cells and waste as it constantly regenerates new healthy cells (autophagy), but excess toxins and nutrient deficiency can impede this important process.

- Emerging research shows that enzyme therapy can help restore autophagy and reverse the health conditions caused by its breakdown.

- Metabolic therapies that utilize enzymes, detoxification, and diet are proving to be even more effective at restoring autophagy.

- Comprehensive immunotherapeutic protocols like those offered at the Issels Clinic utilize enzymes, oxygen, energy, detoxification, homeopathy, nutrition, and more to restore optimal health.

- Supplementing daily with proteolytic enzymes is a great way to prevent autophagic breakdown and the formation of chronic illness.

- Teaching your body to rely on fats rather than carbohydrates for energy (restricted ketogenic diet) can help starve cancer cells.

- Intermittent fasting can also help promote a normalized state of autophagy.

A FINAL WORD

*T*hank you for reading this book. I sincerely hope that it has given you both ammunition and hope. God willing, the day will come when the general public has free access to all natural cancer therapies and advanced medicine is embraced by all practitioners.

It is my sincere desire that this book has enabled you to realize that cancer does not have to be a death sentence. There is always hope. And I trust that this book has made it abundantly clear that you *do* have natural alternatives to the "Big Three"—chemotherapy, radiation, and surgery—although the alternatives may not have the stamp of approval of the cancer industry. Hopefully, you now realize you do *not* have to poison, slash, or burn your body.

A word of caution: *beware of wolves in sheep's clothing!* Hospitals and other providers that offer so-called "nutrition-based" or "holistic" or "integrated" programs often are only paying lip service to patients' requests for natural cancer treatments, just to get them in the door. However, once you're there, they frequently will try to convince you that the conventional treatments are your only hope. You know better. How you treat *your* cancer is *your* choice.

I leave you with the words of Dr. Martin Luther King, Jr.:

"The ultimate measure of a man is not where he stands in moments of comfort and convenience, but where he stands at a time of challenge and controversy."

ENDNOTES

Introduction

1   American Cancer Society, *Cancer Facts and Figures 2015* (Atlanta: American Cancer Society, 2015).

Chapter 1: Hippocrates, Jenner, and Pasteur: Medicine's Beginnings

1   Yapijakis, Christos, "Hippocrates of Kos, the father of clinical medicine, and Asclepiades of Bithynia, the father of molecular medicine," *In Vivo*, 2009 Jul–Aug;23(4):507–14. http://iv.iiarjournals.org/content/23/4/507.full.pdf+html.

2   *The Genuine Works of Hippocrates*, tr. Francis Adams (London: The Sydenham Society, 1849), 360.

3   "Greek Medicine." History of Medicine Division, National Library of Medicine, National Institutes of Health. https://www.nlm.nih.gov/hmd/greek/greek_oath.html.

4   Yapijakis, "Hippocrates of Kos."

5   Ibid.

6   "The Hippocratic Oath Today," *Nova*, March 27, 2001. http://www.pbs.org/wgbh/nova/body/hippocratic-oath-today.html.

7   "Contagion: Historical Views of Diseases and Epidemics," Harvard University Library, Open Collections Program. http://ocp.hul.harvard.edu/contagion/germtheory.html.

8   "Dr. Jenner," http://www.jennermuseum.com/dr-jenner.html.

9   Greenberg, Steven, "A Concise History of Immunology." http://www.columbia.edu/itc/hs/medical/pathophys/immunology/readings/ConciseHistoryImmunology.pdf.

10 Hammarsten, J. F. et al., "Who discovered smallpox vaccination? Edward Jenner or Benjamin Jesty?" *Transactions of the American Clinical and Climatological Association*, 1979;90:44–55. http://www.ncbi.nlm.nih.gov/pmc/articles/PMC2279376/pdf/tacca00099-0087.pdf.

11   Bushak, Lecia, "A Brief History of Vaccines: From Medieval Chinese 'Variolation' to Modern Vaccination," MedicalDaily.com, March 21, 2016.

12   Barnett, Brendon, "Louis Pasteur Biography and Timeline," Pasteur Brewing. http://www.pasteurbrewing.com/biography/biography/history-of-louis-pasteur/78.html.

13   "Louis Pasteur," Biography.com. http://www.biography.com/people/louis-pasteur-9434402.

14   Holsinger, V. H., et al, "Milk pasteurization and safety: a brief history and update," *Revue Scientifique el Technique* (International Office of Epizootics), 1997;16(2):441–51. http://www.oie.int/doc/ged/d9152.pdf.

15   Pearson, R. B., *Pasteur: Plagiarist, Impostor: The Germ Theory Exploded*, 1942. http://www.mnwelldir.org/docs/history/biographies/Bechamp-or-Pasteur.pdf.

16   Garko, M. G., "The terrain within: A naturalistic way to think about and practice good health and wellness," *Health and Wellness Monthly*. Retrieved June 28, 2016, from www.letstalknutrition.com.

17   Ibid.

18   Schultz, Myron, "Rudolph Virchow," *Emerging Infectious Diseases*, 2008;14(9):1480–81. http://www.ncbi.nlm.nih.gov/pmc/articles/PMC2603088/.

19   Leon, Anthony Raphael, *Digestion Takes Precedence over Disease* (Indianapolis: Dog Ear Publishing 2008), 79.

20   Lam, Michael, "Cancer and Biological Terrain," Dr.Lam.com. https://www.drlam.com/blog/cancer-and-biological-terrain/411/.

Chapter 2: The Flexner Report: Big Oil's Takeover of Medicine

1   Beck, Andrew H., "The Flexner Report and the Standardization of American Medical Education," *Journal of the American Medical Association*, 2004 May;291(17). http://hsc.unm.edu/community/toolkit/docs/postflexner.pdf.

2   Duffy, Thomas P., "The Flexner Report—100 Years Later," *Yale Journal of Biology and Medicine*, 2011 Sept.;84(3):269–76. http://www.ncbi.nlm.nih.gov/pmc/articles/PMC3178858/.

3   Ibid.

4   Ibid.

5   Zaidi, Shabih et al., *Teaching and Learning Methods in Medicine* (New York: Springer, 2015), 41.

6   Flexner, Abraham, "Medical Education in the United States and Canada: A Report to the Carnegie Foundation for the Advancement of Teaching," 1910, Introduction, xiv. http://archive.carnegiefoundation.org/pdfs/elibrary/Carnegie_Flexner_Report.pdf.

7   Duffy, "The Flexner Report."

8   Ibid.

9   *History of Royal R. Rife, Jr. (and the Rife Ray Machine)*, DFE Research, 2005. http://www.dfe.net/RifeHist.html.

10   "Who was this man? Why is the drug industry so afraid of him? Royal Raymond Rife," Hidden Mysteries: The Health Archive. http://www.hiddenmysteries.org/health/unbelievable/rife.html.

11   Walters, Richard, "Hoxsey's Herbs Heal Cancers, Red Clover, Burdock Root, others offer track record of success: AMA, NCI, FDA Suppressed Treatment," *The Herb Quarterly*, 1994. http://www.rubysemporium.org/hoxseysherbs.html.

12   Fitzgerald, Benedict, "A Report to the Senate Interstate Commerce Committee on the Need for Investigation of Cancer Research Organizations," *Congressional Record*, 1953:A5350. http://www.newmediaexplorer.org/chris/Fitzgerald%20Report%201953.pdf.

13   Agocs, Steve, "Chiropractic's Fight for Survival," *AMA Journal of Ethics*, 2011;13(6):384–88. http://journalofethics.ama-assn.org/2011/06/mhst1-1106.html.

14   Keating, Joseph Jr., "One Hundred Years Ago in Chiropractic: The Long Trail of Persecution and Prosecution," *Dynamic Chiropractic: The Chiropractic News Source*, 2005. http://www.dynamicchiropractic.com/mpacms/dc/article.php?id=50430.

15   Getzendanner, S., "Permanent injunction order against AMA," *Journal of the American Medical Association,* 1988;259(1):81. http://jama.jamanetwork.com/article.aspx?articleid=370078.

Chapter 3: Smoke and Mirrors

1   Bernays, Edward L., *Propaganda* (New York: Ig Publishing, 1928), 39.

2   Gunderman, Richard, "The manipulation of the American mind—Edward Bernays and the birth of public relations," Phys.org, 2015. http://phys.org/news/2015-07-american-mindedward-bernays-birth.html.

3   Meadowns, Michelle, "Promoting Safe and Effective Drugs for 100 Years," *FDA Consumer,* January–February 2006.

4   López-Muñoz, F., "The pharmaceutical industry and the German National Socialist Regime: I.G. Farben and pharmacological research," *Journal of Clinical Pharmacology and Therapeutics*, 2009 Feb.;34(1):67–77. http://www.ncbi.nlm.nih.gov/pubmed/19125905.

5   Frunzi, Johnathan, "From Weapon to Wonder Drug," *The Hospitalist,* 2007. http://www.the-hospitalist.org/article/from-weapon-to-wonder-drug/?singlepage=1.

Chapter 4: Forced Vaccines? Forced Chemo? Medicine at Gunpoint

1   Gaffney, Alexander, "FDA Publishes All User Fee Rates for Fiscal Year 2014," *Regulatory Affairs Professionals Society,* August 1, 2013. http://www.raps.org/focus-online/news/news-article-view/article/3876/.

2   Herper, Matthew, "The Cost of Creating a New Drug Now $5 Billion, Pushing Big Pharma To Change," *Forbes*, August 11, 2013. http://www.forbes.com/sites/matthewherper/2013/08/11/how-the-staggering-cost-of-inventing-new-drugs-is-shaping-the-future-of-medicine/.

3   Ji, Sayer, "Why the Law Forbids the Medicinal Use of Natural Substances," GreenMedInfo, 2012. http://www.greenmedinfo.com/blog/why-law-forbids-medicinal-use-natural-substances

4   "Laws, Regulations, Policies and Procedures for Drug Applications," U.S. Food and Drug Administration. http://www.fda.gov/Drugs/DevelopmentApprovalProcess/ucm090410.htm.

5   Mercola, Joseph, "The FDA Exposed," Mercola.com. http://www.mercola.com/downloads/bonus/the-FDA-exposed/default.aspx.

6   Wile, Anthony, "Dr. Andrew Wakefield on the Autism/Vaccine Controversy and His Ongoing Professional Persecution," *The Daily Bell*, 2010. http://www.thedailybell.com/asset-protection-strategies/anthony-wile-dr-andrew-wakefield-on-the-autismvaccine-controversy-and-his-ongoing-professional-persecution/.

7   Richardson, Dawn, "The Fallout from California SB277: What Happens Next?" National Vaccine Information Center, August 5, 2015. http://www.nvic.org/nvic-vaccine-news/august-2015/sb277-fallout-what-happens-next.aspx.

8   Lynne, Diana, "Newborn Vaccinated over Parents' Objections," WorldNetDaily, June 18, 2003. http://www.wnd.com/2003/06/19338/.

9   Andrews, Michelle, "Some Doctors Refuse to Treat Kids Who Have Not Been Immunized," *Kaiser Health News*, September 26, 2011. http://khn.org/news/michelle-andrews-on-kids-vaccines-and-refusal/.

10   Linderman, Curt Sr., "Doctor Calls Police, Child Services on Mother Who Refuses to Vaccinate Son," *Infowars*, January 17, 2012. http://www.infowars.com/doctor-calls-police-child-services-on-mother-who-refuses-to-vaccinate-son/.

11   Matturri, L., et al., "Sudden Infant Death Following Hexavalent Vaccination: A Neuropathologic Study," *Current Medicinal Chemistry*, 2014 Mar;21(7):941–46. http://www.eurekaselect.com/115921/article.

12   Buttram, Harold E., "Shaken Baby Syndrome or Vaccine-Induced Encephalitis?" *Journal of American Physicians and Surgeons*, 2001;6(3):83–89. http://www.jpands.org/hacienda/buttram.html.

13   Al-Bayati, Mohammed Ali, "Analysis of Causes That Led to Baby Robert Benjamin Quirello's Respiratory Arrest and Death in August of 2000," 2004. http://truthinjustice.org/Baby-Robert-Report-final-2004.doc.

14   Johnson, Avery, "Vaccine Makers Enjoy Immunity," *The Wall Street Journal*, February 23, 2009. http://www.wsj.com/articles/SB123535050056344903.

15   "State Law & Vaccine Requirements," National Vaccine Information

Center. http://www.nvic.org/vaccine-laws/state-vaccine-requirements. aspx.

16 *Vaxxed: From Cover-Up to Catastrophe*, 2016. http://www. vaxxedthemovie.com.

17 Rappoport, Jon, "The vaccine film Robert De Niro won't let his audience see," *Jon Rappoport's Blog*, 2016. https://jonrappoport.wordpress. com/2016/03/27/the-vaccine-film-robert-deniro-wont-let-his-audience-see/.

18 Miller, Doug, "'Vaxxed' pulled from Houston's International Film Fest," KHOU, 2016. http://www.khou.com/entertainment/vaxxed-pulled-from-houstons-international-film-fest/125142297.

19 Yang, Guodong, et al., "Chemotherapy not only enriches but also induces cancer stem cells," *Biosciences Hypotheses*, 2009;2(6):393–95. http:// www.sciencedirect.com/science/article/pii/S1756239209001323.

20 Periyakoil, Vyjeyanthi S. et al., "Do Unto Others: Doctors' Personal End-of-Life Resuscitation Preferences and Their Attitudes toward Advance Directives," *PLOS One*, 2014 May;9(5):e98246. http://journals. plos.org/plosone/article?id=10.1371/journal.pone.0098246.

21 Innes, Emma, "Most doctors who were terminally ill would AVOID aggressive treatment," *The Daily Mail*, May 30, 2014. http://www. dailymail.co.uk/health/article-2643751/Most-doctors-terminally-ill-AVOID-aggressive-treatments-chemotherapy-despite-recommending-patients.html.

22 Smith, Thomas J., et al., "Would Oncologists Want Chemotherapy if They Had Non-Small-Cell Lung Cancer?" *Oncology*, March 1, 1998. http://www.cancernetwork.com/articles/would-oncologists-want-chemotherapy-if-they-had-non-small-cell-lung-cancer.

23 Lind, S. E., et al., "Oncologists vary in their willingness to undertake anti-cancer therapies," *British Journal of Cancer*, 1991;64:391–95. http://www.ncbi.nlm.nih.gov/pmc/articles/PMC1977523/pdf/brjcancer00072-0193.pdf.

24 Ellis, Rehema, "Cancer docs profit from chemotherapy drugs," NBC News, 2006. http://www.nbcnews.com/id/14944098/ns/nbc_nightly_news_with_brian_williams/t/cancer-docs-profit-chemotherapy-drugs/.

25 Morgan, G., et al., "The contribution of cytotoxic chemotherapy to 5-year survival in adult malignancies," *Journal of Clinical Oncology*, 2004 Dec;16(8):549–60. http://www.ncbi.nlm.nih.gov/ pubmed/15630849.

26 Bollinger, Ty, "The Medical Kidnapping of Cassandra C: Exclusive TTAC Interview (Video)," *The Truth About Cancer*. https://thetruthaboutcancer.com/the-medical-kidnapping-of-cassandra-c/.

27 Mercola, Joseph, "Two Words You Should Never Utter to Your Doctor," Mercola.com, 2011. http://articles.mercola.com/sites/articles/ archive/2011/09/24/jim-navarro-featured-in-cut-poison-burn.aspx.

28   *Kid Against Chemo*. http://kidagainstchemo.wix.com/kidagainstchemo.

Chapter 5: Cancer Basics and Statistics

1   Bianconi, Eva et al., "An estimation of the number of cells in the human body," *Annals of Human Biology*, 2013;6(40):463–71. http://www.tandfonline.com/doi/full/10.3109/03014460.2013.807878.

2   Bollinger, Ty, "What is Cancer?" *Cancer Truth*, 2011. http://www.cancertruth.net/test-2/#sthash.yZ5LxFTa.LBFrejSD.dpbs.

3   Jurasunas, Serge, "The Clinical Evidence of Cellular Respiration to Target Cancer." http://www.sergejurasunas.com/index.php?option=com_content&view=article&id=70:the-clinical-evidence-of-cellular-respiration-to-target-cancer&catid=21:clinical-strategy.

4   Warburg, Otto, "The Prime Cause and Prevention of Cancer," lecture delivered at the meeting of the Nobel-Laureates on June 30, 1966, at Lindau, Lake Constance, Germany.

5   Jurasunas, "The Clinical Evidence of Cellular Respiration to Target Cancer."

6   Macrae, Fiona, "Cancer 'is purely man-made' say scientists after finding almost no trace of disease in Egyptian mummies," *The Daily Mail*, October 15, 2010. http://www.dailymail.co.uk/sciencetech/article-1320507/Cancer-purely-man-say-scientists-finding-trace-disease-Egyptian-mummies.html.

7   "Cancer Statistics," National Cancer Institute. http://www.cancer.gov/about-cancer/what-is-cancer/statistics.

8   Dinse, G. E., et al., "Unexplained increases in cancer incidence in the United States from 1975 to 1994," *Annual Review of Public Health*, 1999;20:173–209. http://www.ncbi.nlm.nih.gov/pubmed/10352856.

9   Greenlee, Robert T., et al., "Cancer statistics, 2000," *CA: A Cancer Journal for Clinicians*, 2008;50(1):7–33. http://onlinelibrary.wiley.com/doi/10.3322/canjclin.50.1.7/full.

10   "Statistics and General Facts," Breast Cancer Action. http://archive.bcaction.org/index.php?page=statistics-and-general-facts.

11   Brawley, O. W., "Trends in prostate cancer in the United States," *Journal of the National Cancer Institute Monographs*, 2012 Dec;2012(45):152–56. http://www.ncbi.nlm.nih.gov/pubmed/23271766.

12   Elkins, Chris, "How Much Cancer Costs," DrugWatch, 2015. https://www.drugwatch.com/2015/10/07/cost-of-cancer/.

13   Mariotto, A.B., et al., "Projections of the Cost of Cancer Care in the United States: 2010–2020," *Journal of the National Cancer Institute*, 2011;103(2).

14   Howard, David H., "Pricing in the Market for Anticancer Drugs," *Journal of Economic Perspectives*, 2015;29(1):139–162.

15   Hanly, P., Soerjomataram, I., and Sharp, L., "Measuring the societal

burden of cancer: The cost of lost productivity due to premature cancer-related mortality in Europe," *International Journal of Cancer*, 2014;136(4):136–145.

16   Bollyky, Thomas, "Why Chemotherapy That Costs $70,000 in the U.S. Costs $2,500 in India," *The Atlantic*, April 10, 2013. http://www.the-atlantic.com/health/archive/2013/04/why-chemotherapy-that-costs-70-000-in-the-us-costs-2-500-in-india/274847/.

17   Jaffe, Susan, "USA grapples with high drug costs," *The Lancet*, 2015 Nov;386(10009):2127–28. http://thelancet.com/journals/lancet/artic-le/PIIS0140-6736(15)01098-3/fulltext.

18   Albright, Logan, "Blame Government for High Drug Prices," *Freedom-Works*, September 23, 2015.

Chapter 6: Cancer Causes . . . Is Cancer Genetic?

1   Humphries, Courtney, "Which types of cancer are hereditary?" Boston. com, January 3, 2011. http://archive.boston.com/lifestyle/health/arti-cles/2011/01/03/cancer_isnt_hereditary_but_susceptibility_to_it_is/.

2   Reuben, Suzanne H., *Reducing Environmental Cancer Risk: What We Can Do Now* (U.S. Department of Health and Human Services, 2010).

3   Unsworth, John, "History of Pesticide Use," International Union of Pure and Applied Chemistry, 2010. http://agrochemicals.iupac.org/index. php?option=com_sobi2&sobi2Task=sobi2Details&catid=3&sobi-2Id=31.

4   Ibid.

5   "Cancer," Pesticide Action Network North America. http://www.panna. org/human-health-harms/cancer.

6   Majewski, M. S., et al., "Pesticides in Mississippi air and rain: a comparison between 1995 and 2007," *Environmental Toxicology Chemistry*, 2014 Jun;33(6):1283–93. https://www.ncbi.nlm.nih.gov/pubmed/24549493.

7   Reuben, *Reducing Environmental Cancer Risk*, 45.

8   "Genetically Modified Foods," American Academy of Environmental Medicine. http://www.aaemonline.org/gmo.php.

9   "Cancer-Causing Substances in the Environment," National Cancer Institute. http://www.cancer.gov/about-cancer/causes-prevention/risk/substances.

10   Bennett, J. W., and Klich, M., "Mycotoxins," *Clinical Microbiology Reviews*, 2003, Jul;16(3):497–516. http://www.ncbi.nlm.nih.gov/pmc/articles/PMC164220/.

11   "Vaccine Excipient & Media Summary: Excipients Included in U.S. Vaccines, by Vaccine," *Epidemiology and Prevention of Vaccine-Preventable Diseases* (U.S. Centers for Disease Control and Prevention, 2015), Appendix B. http://www.cdc.gov/vaccines/pubs/pinkbook/downloads/

appendices/B/excipient-table-2.pdf.

12   "Formaldehyde in Vaccines: A DNA Adduct?," VacTruth.com, February 7, 2012. http://vactruth.com/2012/02/07/formaldehyde-vaccines-dna-adduct/.

13   Boffetta, P., et al., "Carcinogenicity of mercury and mercury compounds," *Scandinavian Journal of Work, Environment & Health*, 1993, Feb;19(1):1–7. http://www.ncbi.nlm.nih.gov/pubmed/8465166.

14   "Electromagnetic fields and public health: mobile phones," World Health Organization, 2014. http://www.who.int/mediacentre/factsheets/fs193/en/.

15   Blank, Martin, "Caution: Cell Phone Use Can Double Your Risk of Getting a Brain Tumor," Mercola.com, accessed June 28, 2016.

16   Alexiou, George A., "Mobile phone use and risk for intracranial tumors," *Journal of Negative Results in BioMedicine*, 2015, Dec;14:23. http://jnrbm.biomedcentral.com/articles/10.1186/s12952-015-0043-7.

17   Connett, Paul, et al., "Revisiting the Fluoride-Osteosarcoma connection in the context of Elise Bassin's findings: Part II," submitted to the NRC review panel on the Toxicology of Fluoride in Water, April 8, 2005.

18   Bassin, E. B., et al., "Age-specific fluoride exposure in drinking water and osteosarcoma (United States), *Cancer, Causes & Control*, 2006, May;17(4):421–28. http://www.ncbi.nlm.nih.gov/pubmed/16596294.

19   "Cancer," Fluoride Action Network. http://fluoridealert.org/issues/health/cancer/.

20   Dhimolea, Eugen, et al., "Prenatal Exposure to BPA Alters the Epigenome of the Rat Mammary Gland and Increases the Propensity to Neoplastic Development," *PLOS One*, 2014, Jul;9(7):e99800. http://www.environmentalhealthnews.org/ehs/news/pdf-links-2014/pone%200099800%20final.pdf.

21   "Adverse Health Effects of Plastics," Ecology Center. http://ecologycenter.org/factsheets/adverse-health-effects-of-plastics/.

22   MacKenzie, Margaret, "Chemtrails Linked to Cancer, Scientists Say," Wyoming Institute of Technology, 2014. http://witscience.org/chemtrails-linked-cancer-scientists-say/.

23   Nierenberg, Cari, "New Health Warning Explained: How Processed Meat is Linked to Cancer," *LiveScience*, 2015. http://www.livescience.com/52651-red-meat-cancer-warning-explained.html.

Chapter 7: Detection "Dos" and "Don'ts"

1   "Do Mammograms Cause Cancer?" Dr.Axe.com. http://draxe.com/mammograms-cause-cancer/.

2   Hubbard, Sylvia Booth, "Can Mammograms Spread Cancer?" Newsmax, October 1, 2015. http://www.newsmax.com/Health/Headline/mammograms-spread-cancer-Russell-Blaylock/2015/10/01/

id/694339/.

3   Mercola, Joseph, "Your Greatest Weapon Against Breast Cancer (Not Mammograms)," Mercola.com, March 3, 2012. http://articles.mercola.com/sites/articles/archive/2012/03/03/experts-say-avoid-mammograms.aspx.

4   "Why most men don't need a PSA test for prostate cancer: Much of what you've heard about how to prevent, detect, and treat this common cancer is wrong," *Consumer Reports*, February 2015. http://www.consumerreports.org/cro/news/2015/02/most-men-dont-need-a-psa-test-for-prostate-cancer/index.htm.

5   Ji, Sayer, "The Dark Side of Breast Cancer (Un)Awareness Month," GreenMedInfo, 2012. http://www.greenmedinfo.com/blog/dark-side-breast-cancer-unawareness-month.

6   Northrup, Christiane, "Best Breast Test: The Promise of Thermography," Dr.Northrup.com. http://www.drnorthrup.com/best-breast-test/.

7   Smith, Tim, "The AMAS Test: An Alternative to Nagalase Testing," *The GcMAF Book (2.0)*, 2010. http://gcmaf.timsmithmd.com/book/chapter/20/.

8   Oncolab AMAS Testing. http://www.oncolabinc.com/patients.html.

9   "HCG Urine Immunoassay: A safe, cost-effective, non-invasive, accurate screening test for Cancer," Navarro Medical Clinic. http://www.navarromedicalclinic.com/index.php.

10   Cagan, Michele, "The one cancer test that could save your life . . . if only you knew about it," *Health Sciences Institute*, 2013 Apr;17(8):2,6. http://www.cancercenterforhealing.com/wp-content/uploads/2013/12/Oncoblot-report.pdf?171766.

11   "Blood Test for Cancer," ONCOblot Labs. http://oncoblotlabs.com/how-it-works/.

12   Alegre, Melissa M., et al., "Thymidine Kinase 1: A Universal Marker for Cancer," *Cancer and Clinical Oncology*, 2013 May;2(1). http://www.ccsenet.org/journal/index.php/cco/article/download/26281/16499&usg=AFQjCNHzbbRvsvszXFQ2oDiiVc5KQt-4J3Q&cad=rja

13   O'Neill, Kim L., et al., "Thymidine kinase: diagnostic and prognostic potential," *Expert Review of Molecular Diagnostics*, 2001:1(4). http://www.reddrop.com/wp-content/uploads/2013/03/TK-review.pdf.

14   Alegre, Melissa M., et al., "Serum Detection of Thymidine Kinase 1 as a Means of Early Detection of Lung Cancer," *Anticancer Research*, 2014;34:2145–52. http://www.iiar-anticancer.org/openAR/journals/index.php/anticancer/article/download/493/486&usg=AFQjCNEg-jQ4T9iPQ-POOgW2oy07E4ofG8A&sig2=SZw203ZuJXDXKrmjC-Blzvg&bvm=bv.119745492,d.eWE.

15   Smith, "The AMAS Test."

16   Giandomenico, Nicol, "What is Nagalase?" Dr. Klinghardt, 2015. http://drklinghardt.com/what-is-nagalase-by-dr-nicol-giandomenico/.

17   The Hilu Institute, Foundation for Alternative and Integrative Medicine. http://www.faim.org/the-hilu-institute.

Chapter 8: How Can I Prevent Cancer?

1   Health Creation: A life energy management approach to vitality, health and wellbeing. http://www.healthcreation.co.uk.

2   Daniel, Rosy, and Ellis, Rachel, *The Cancer Prevention Book* (New York: Simon & Schuster, 2002), 22.

3   Seidl, L. G., "The value of spiritual health," *Health Progress*, 1993 Sep;74(7):48–50. http://www.ncbi.nlm.nih.gov/pubmed/10127982.

4   Breast Cancer Conqueror, "The 7 Essentials System." http://breastcancerconqueror.com/about/7-essentials/.

5   Sears, Margaret E., et al., "Arsenic, Cadmium, Lead, and Mercury in Sweat: A Systematic Review," *Journal of Environmental and Public Health*, 2012 Feb;184745. http://www.ncbi.nlm.nih.gov/pmc/articles/PMC3312275/

6   "Exercise intensity: How to measure it," Mayo Clinic. http://www.mayoclinic.org/healthy-lifestyle/fitness/in-depth/exercise-intensity/art-20046887

7   "Aerobic Exercise Intensity and Target Heart Rate," HPM Corporation. http://www.hanford.gov/health/?page=112.

8   Walsh, Neil P., and Oliver, Samuel J., "Exercise, immune function and respiratory infection: An update on the influence of training and environmental stress," *Immunology and Cell Biology*, 2016 Feb;94(2):132–39. http://www.nature.com/icb/journal/v94/n2/full/icb201599a.html.

9   "Trans Fatty Acids," University of Iowa Hospitals and Clinics. http://www.news-releases.uiowa.edu/2003/september/090803trans-fatty-acids.html.

10   Bunim, Juliana, "Societal control of sugar essential to ease public health burden," UCSF News Center, February 1, 2012; and "The top 10 causes of death," World Health Organization, 2014. http://www.who.int/mediacentre/factsheets/fs310/en/.

11   Sircus, Mark, "Cancer & Sugar—Strategy for Selective Starvation of Cancer," GreenMedInfo, 2013. http://www.greenmedinfo.com/blog/cancer-sugar-strategy-selective-starvation-cancer.

12   University of Utah Health Science, "Does Sugar Feed Cancer?" *ScienceDaily*, 2009. https://www.sciencedaily.com/releases/2009/08/090817184539.htm.

13   "Names of ingredients that contain processed free glutamic acid (MSG)," Truth in Labeling, 2014. http://www.truthinlabeling.org/hiddensources.html.

14   Gennet, Robbie, "Donald Rumsfeld and the Strange History of

Aspartame," *The Huffington Post,* January 26, 2011. http://www.huff-ingtonpost.com/robbie-gennet/donald-rumsfeld-and-the-s_b_805581.html.

15   Mercola, Joseph, "Aspartame: By Far the Most Dangerous Substance Added to Most Foods Today," Mercola.com, November 6, 2011. http://articles.mercola.com/sites/articles/archive/2011/11/06/aspartame-most-dangerous-substance-added-to-food.aspx.

16   "10 Reasons to Avoid GMOs," Institute for Responsible Technology. http://responsibletechnology.org/10-reasons-to-avoid-gmos/.

17   GMOEvidence. http://www.gmoevidence.com.

18   Smith, Jeffrey, "Health Risks," Institute for Responsible Technology. http://responsibletechnology.org/gmo-education/health-risks/.

19   Ibid.

20   "Healthy Home Tips: Tip 6—Skip the Non-Stick to Avoid the Dangers of Teflon," The Environmental Working Group. http://www.ewg.org/research/healthy-home-tips/tip-6-skip-non-stick-avoid-dangers-teflon.

21   Group, Edward, "Why You Should Never Microwave Your Food," Global Healing Center, 2015. http://www.globalhealingcenter.com/natural-health/why-you-should-never-microwave-your-food/.

22   Mercola, Joseph, "The Little-Known Secrets about Bleached Flour," Mercola.com, March 26, 2009. http://articles.mercola.com/sites/articles/archive/2009/03/26/The-Little-Known-Secrets-about-Bleached-Flour.aspx.

23   "All 48 Fruits and Vegetables with Pesticide Residue Data," The Environmental Working Group. https://www.ewg.org/foodnews/list.php.

24   "EWG's Skin Deep Cosmetics Database," The Environmental Working Group. http://www.ewg.org/skindeep/.

25   Wong, William, "Soy: The Poison Seed," Totality of Being. http://www.totalityofbeing.com/FramelessPages/Articles/SoyPoison.htm.

26   "Cancer," Fluoride Action Network. http://fluoridealert.org/issues/health/cancer/.

27   Wong, Matthew, et al., "Organochlorine Pesticide Toxicity," Medscape, 2015. http://emedicine.medscape.com/article/815051-overview.

28   Woollams, Chris, "The Rainbow Diet." http://www.the-rainbow-diet.com/pages/the-research/2.

29   David, Yair et al., "Water Intake and Cancer Prevention," *Journal of Clinical Oncology,* 2004 Jan;22(2):383–85. http://jco.ascopubs.org/content/22/2/383.1.full.

30   Ayas, N. T., et al., "A prospective study of self-reported sleep duration and incident diabetes in women," *Diabetes Care,* 2003 Feb;26(2):380–84. http://www.ncbi.nlm.nih.gov/pubmed/12547866?dopt=Abstract.

31   O'Shea, Tim, "Enzymes: The Key to Longevity," Spirit of Health. http://www.spiritofhealthkc.com/portfolio/enzymes-the-key-to-longevity/.

Chapter 9: Herbal Remedies, Detoxification, and Diet

1   Robbins, John, *Reclaiming Our Health: Exploding the Medical Myth and Embracing the Source of True Healing* (Tiburon, CA: H. J. Kramer, 1998), 272.

2   Resperin's Original Caisse Formula Tea, Resperin Canada Limited. http://www.resperin.ca.

3   The Rene Caisse Room, Rene Caisse Tea. http://renecaissetea.com/the-rene-caisse-room/.

4   "Burdock," University of Maryland Medical Center. http://umm.edu/health/medical/altmed/herb/burdock.

5   Havasi, Peter, *Education of Cancer Healing Vol. IV: Crusaders* (Lulu.com, 2012), 90.

6   Barron, Jon, "Sheep Sorrel: A Rich Source of Vitamin C, E, Beta-Carotene, and Other Carotenoids," Baseline of Health Foundation. http://jonbarron.org/herbal-library/herbs/sheep-sorrel.

7   Grattan, Bruce J., Jr., "Plant Sterols as Anticancer Nutrients: Evidence for Their Role in Breast Cancer," *Nutrients,* 2013;5(2), 359–387.

8   Cai, J., et al., "Feasibility evaluation of emodin (rhubarb extract) as an inhibitor of pancreatic cancer cell proliferation in vitro," *Journal of Parenteral and Enteral Nutrition,* 2008 Mar–Apr;32(2):190–96. http://www.ncbi.nlm.nih.gov/pubmed/18407913.

9   Ausubel, Kenny, "Tempest in a Tonic Bottle: A Bunch of Weeds?" *HerbalGram,* 2000;49:32–43, American Botanical Council. http://cms.herbalgram.org/herbalgram/issue49/article2270.html?ts=1461448105&signature=ae7086ca20e4b604d513e0fc25ed1454.

10   Urbaniak, Eva, "Hoxsey: A Winning Formula Against Cancer," Dr. Eva Online. http://www.docevaonline.com/articles/hoxsey.html.

11   De Lago, E., et al., "Acyl-based anandamide uptake inhibitors cause rapid toxicity to C6 glioma cells at pharmacologically relevant concentrations," *Journal of Neurochemistry,* 2006 Oct;99(2):677–88. http://www.ncbi.nlm.nih.gov/pubmed/16899063.

12   Preet, A., et al., "Delta9-Tetrahydrocannabinol inhibits epithelial growth factor-induced lung cancer cell migration *in vitro* as well as its growth and metastasis *in vivo*," *Oncogene,* 2008 Jan;27(3):339–46. http://www.nature.com/onc/journal/v27/n3/abs/1210641a.html.

13   Leelawat, S., et al., "The dual effects of delta(9)-tetrahydrocannabinol on cholangiocarcinoma cells: anti-invasion activity at low concentration and apoptosis induction at high concentration," *Cancer Investigation,* 2010 May;28(4):357–63. https://www.ncbi.nlm.nih.gov/pubmed/19916793.

14   Glodde, N., et al., "Differential role of cannabinoids in the pathogenesis of skin cancer," *Life Science,* 2015 Oct 1;138:35–40. https://www.ncbi.nlm.nih.gov/pubmed/25921771.

15   Lombard, C., et al., "Targeting cannabinoid receptors to treat leukemia: role of cross-talk between extrinsic and intrinsic pathways in Delta9-tetrahydrocannabinol (THC)-induced apoptosis of Jurkat cells," *Leukemia Research*, 2005 Aug;29(8):915–22. https://www.ncbi.nlm.nih.gov/pubmed/15978942.

16   Nelson, Steven, "Study: Cannabis Compounds Can Kill Cancer Cells." *U.S. News & World Report*, October 24, 2013. http://www.usnews.com/news/articles/2013/10/24/study-cannabis-compounds-can-kill-cancer-cells.

17   United Patients Group, "THC, THCA, CBD, CBC, CBN: Some of the Chemicals in Cannabis." http://www.unitedpatientsgroup.com/blog/2014/04/11/thc-thca-cbd-cbn-the-chemicals-in-cannabis/.

18   United Patients Group, "THC, THCA, CBD, CBC, CBN."

19   Young, Francis L., "Opinion and Recommended Ruling, Findings of Fact, Conclusions of Law and Decision of Administrative Law Judge," 1988. http://www.ccguide.org/young88.php.

20   "5 Reasons to Juice Your Cannabis," Leaf Science, 2014. http://www.leafscience.com/2014/07/18/5-reasons-juice-cannabis/.

21   United Patients Group, "Juicing Cannabis: The Freshest Medicine?" 2014. http://www.unitedpatientsgroup.com/blog/2014/03/28/juicing-cannabis-the-freshest-medicine/.

22   Ibid.

23   Simpson, Rick, "Phoenix Tears." http://phoenixtears.ca.

24   "24 Legal Medical Marijuana States and D.C.," ProCon.org, 2016. http://medicalmarijuana.procon.org/view.resource.php?resourceID=000881.

25   Smith, Carol, "Trevor Smith's Story: How He Beat Bladder Cancer Naturally with Cannabis Oil," Cure Your Own Cancer, 2014. http://www.cureyourowncancer.org/trevor-smiths-story-how-he-beat-bladder-cancer-naturally-with-cannabis-oil.html.

26   Barron, Jon, "Blood Cleansing Herbs & Supplements," Baseline of Health Foundation, 2014. http://jonbarron.org/blood-cleansing/cleansing-your-blood.

27   The Gerson Institute. https://gerson.org/gerpress/gerson-clinic-mexico/.

28   The Gerson Institute. http://gerson.org/gerpress/gerson-health-centre/.

29   The Gerson Institute. http://gerson.org/gerpress/the-gerson-therapy/.

30   Ji, Sayer, "600 Reasons Turmeric May Be the World's Most Important Herb," GreenMedInfo, 2013. http://www.greenmedinfo.com/blog/600-reasons-turmeric-may-be-worlds-most-important-herb.

31   Mercola, Joseph, "What the Research Really Says About Apple Cider Vinegar," Mercola.com, June 2, 2009. http://articles.mercola.com/sites/articles/archive/2009/06/02/apple-cider-vinegar-hype.aspx.

32   Vitälzym, World Nutrition Inc. http://worldnutrition.net/products/

vitalz⬛m-soft-liquid-gel/.

33 VeganZyme, Global Healing Center. http://www.globalhealingcenter.com/veganzyme.html.

34 Wobenzym N, Garden of Life. http://www.gardenoflife.com/content/product/wobenzym-n/.

35 "Laetrile therapy at Oasis of Hope," Oasis of Hope Hospital. http://www.oasisofhope.com/cancer-treatments-therapies/laetrile/.

Chapter 10: Sound, Light, Electricity, Frequency, and Heat

1 Mead, Nathaniel M., "Benefits of Sunlight: A Bright Spot for Human Health," *Environmental Health Perspectives*, 2008 Apr;116(4):A160–67. http://www.ncbi.nlm.nih.gov/pmc/articles/PMC2290997/.

2 "The Therapy," Sono-Photo Dynamic Therapy. Hope4Cancer Institute. http://www.sonophotodynamictherapy.com/sonophotodynamictherapy_therapy.html.

3 Chakravarty, Subrata, "Trina Hammack, 5-Year Stage 4 Ovarian Cancer Survivor: 'I Beat the Odds,'" Hope4Cancer Institute, 2013. http://www.hope4cancer.com/information/trina-stage-4-ovarian-cancer.html.

4 Chakravarty, Subrata, "Meet Our Hero, Charles Daniel: 7 Years Free of Stage 4 Bladder Cancer," Hope4Cancer Institute, 2015. http://www.hope4cancer.com/information/charles-daniel-stage-4-bladder-cancer.html.

5 Pawluk, William, "Magnetic Field Therapy Introduction," DrPawluk.com. https://www.drpawluk.com/education/introduction-to-magnetic-field-therapy/.

6 Valone, Thomas, *The Future of Energy: An Emerging Science* (Beltsville, MD: Integrity Research Institute, 2009), 28.

7 American Institute of Physics, "Electric Fields Have Potential as a Cancer Treatment," ScienceDaily, 2007. https://www.sciencedaily.com/releases/2007/08/070802100748.htm.

8 Kehr, Webster, "Frequency Generator Protocols for Cancer Stage IV Protocol," Independent Cancer Research Foundation, Inc., 2015. https://www.cancertutor.com/freqgenerators/.

9 Kehr, Webster, "Cellect-Budwig Protocol A Stage IV Cancer Treatment," Independent Cancer Research Foundation, Inc., 2015. https://www.cancertutor.com/cellect_budwig/.

10 Kehr, Webster, "The Plasma-Beck Protocol for Cancer Stage IV Protocol," Independent Cancer Research Foundation, Inc., 2015. https://www.cancertutor.com/plasmabeck/.

11 Healing Water Technology, MRET. http://www.healingwatertechnology.com/index.php.

12   Takata, K., et al., "Aquaporins: water channel proteins of the cell membrane," *Progress in Histochemistry and Cytochemistry*, 2004;39(1):1–83. http://www.ncbi.nlm.nih.gov/pubmed/15242101.

13   MRET Water Activator, Healing Water Technology. http://www.healingwatertechnology.com/order.php.

14   Karbach, Julia, "Phase I clinical trial of Mixed Bacterial Vaccine (Coley's Toxins) in patients with NY-ESO-1 expressing cancers: Immunological effects and clinical activity," *Clinical Cancer Research*, 2012. http://clincancerres.aacrjournals.org/content/early/2012/07/28/1078-0432.CCR-12-1116.full.pdf.

15   Fenn, Alan J., et al., "Improved Localization of Energy Deposition in Adaptive Phased-Array Hyperthermia Treatment of Cancer," *The Lincoln Laboratory Journal,* 1996;9(2).

16   Fassa, Paul, "How Fever Can Cure Cancer," *Natural News*, March 19, 2011.

17   "Overheating Therapy," Rudolf Steiner Health Center, http://www.steinerhealth.org/health/fever-therapy/.

Chapter 11: Bio-Oxidative Therapies

1   Brand, Richard, "Biographical Sketch: Otto Heinrich Warburg, Ph.D., M.D.," *Clinical Orthopaedics and Related Research*, 2010 Nov;468(11):2831–32. http://www.ncbi.nlm.nih.gov/pmc/articles/PMC2947689/.

2   Elvis, A. M., and Ekta, J. S., "Ozone therapy: A clinical review," *Journal of Natural Science, Biology and Medicine*, 2011 Jan–Jun;2(1):66–70. http://www.ncbi.nlm.nih.gov/pmc/articles/PMC3312702/.

3   "The Benefits of Steam Sauna and Ozone," *Health News & Views from Netherspring*, January 27, 2008.

4   "Dr. John Harvey Kellogg—Inventor of Kellogg's Corn Flakes," University of Texas Health Science Center. http://library.uthscsa.edu/2014/05/dr-john-harvey-kellogg-inventor-of-kelloggs-corn-flakes/

5   Kellogg, J. H., *Diphtheria: Its Causes, Prevention, and Proper Treatment* (Battle Creek, MI: Good Health Publishing Co., 1879).

6   "Ozone History & Nikola Tesla," *Ozone Science*, December 27, 2007.

7   Sweet, F., et al., "Ozone selectively inhibits growth of human cancer cells," *Science*, 1980;209:931–933.

8   Farr, Charles, "The Therapeutic Use of Intravenous Hydrogen Peroxide: A Review: Experimental Evidence of Physiological Effect and Clinical Experience," 1986–1987. http://www.foodgrade-hydrogenperoxide.com/sitebuildercontent/sitebuilderfiles/TherapeuticUseOfHPFarr.pdf.

9   Altman, Nathaniel, "Ozone—Oxygen Therapies," Oxygen Healing Therapies. http://www.oxygenhealingtherapies.com/ozone_oxygen_therapies.html.

10   Roguski, James Paul, "The Truth about Food Grade Hydrogen

Peroxide." http://www.foodgrade-hydrogenperoxide.com/sitebuilder-content/sitebuilderfiles/thetruthaboutfghp.pdf.

11   "Oxidative & Alternative Oxygen Therapies," Health and Wellness Foundation. http://www.johnpridgeon.com/yahoo_site_admin/assets/docs/Oxidative_and_Alternative_Oxygen_Therapies.23390533.docx.

12   In Kehr, Webster, "High Dose Intravenous Vitamin C (IVC)," Independent Cancer Research Foundation, Inc., 2015. https://www.cancertutor.com/vitaminc_ivc/.

13   *Vitamin C: Fact Sheet for Health Professionals.* National Institutes of Health: Office of Dietary Supplements. https://ods.od.nih.gov/factsheets/VitaminC-HealthProfessional/.

14   Mikirova, N., et al., "Effect of high-dose intravenous vitamin C on inflammation in cancer patients," *Journal of Translational Medicine*, 2012 Sep 11;10:189. http://www.ncbi.nlm.nih.gov/pubmed/22963460.

15   Levy, Thomas E., "Pulsed intravenous vitamin C (PIVC) therapy," *Health E-Bytes*, July 2003.

Chapter 12: Treating Cancer with Viruses and Essential Oils

1   "10 Healthiest Fermented Foods & Vegetables," DrAxe.com. http://draxe.com/fermented-foods/.

2   Skwarecki, Beth, "Friendly Viruses Protect Us Against Bacteria," *Science*, May 2013. http://www.sciencemag.org/news/2013/05/friendly-viruses-protect-us-against-bacteria.

3   Ledford, Heidi, "Cancer-fighting viruses win approval," *Nature*, 2015 Oct;526(7575). http://www.nature.com/news/cancer-fighting-viruses-win-approval-1.18651.

4   Muceniece, Aina, "New Era in Cancer Treatment," Cancer Virotherapy. http://www.virotherapy.eu.

5   "Exploring Aromatherapy: Aromatherapy is an incredibly vast and rich field," National Association for Holistic Aromatherapy. https://www.naha.org/explore-aromatherapy/about-aromatherapy/what-are-essential-oils/.

6   Tisserand, Robert, "Frankincense Oil and Cancer in Perspective," Tisserand Institute. http://tisserandinstitute.org/frankincense-oil-and-cancer-in-perspective/.

7   Chen, Yingli, et al., "Composition and potential anticancer activities of essential oils obtained from myrrh and frankincense," *Oncology Letters*, 2013 Oct;6(4):1140–46. http://www.ncbi.nlm.nih.gov/pmc/articles/PMC3796379/.

8   Bayala, Bagora, "Anticancer activity of essential oils and their chemical components—a review," *American Journal of Cancer Research*, 2014;4(6):591–607. http://www.ncbi.nlm.nih.gov/pmc/articles/PMC4266698/.

Chapter 13: Enzyme and Metabolic/Mitochondrial Therapy

1   Lee, Jin-A, "Neuronal Autophagy: A Housekeeper or a Fighter in Neuronal Cell Survival?" *Experimental Neurobiology*, 2012 Mar;21(1):1–8. http://www.ncbi.nlm.nih.gov/pmc/articles/PMC3294068/.

2   Watson, James, Giuliano, Vance, "Autophagy—the housekeeper in every cell that fights aging," *AgingSciences: Anti-Aging Firewalls*, 2013. http://www.anti-agingfirewalls.com/2013/04/19/autophagy-the-housekeeper-in-every-cell-that-fights-aging-2/.

3   Mercola, Joseph, "The Metabolic Theory of Cancer and the Key to Cancer Prevention and Recovery," Mercola.com, February 7, 2016.

4   Seyfried, Thomas, et al., "Cancer as a metabolic disease: implications for novel therapeutics," *Carcinogenesis*, 2014 Mar;35(3):515–27. http://www.ncbi.nlm.nih.gov/pmc/articles/PMC3941741/.

5   Goodman, Ira, "Refocusing Our Efforts Against Cancer," *Townsend Letter: The Examiner of Alternative Medicine*, 2015. http://www.townsendletter.com/Nov2015/bk_trip1115.html.

6   Christofferson, Travis, *Tripping Over the Truth: The Return of the Metabolic Theory of Cancer Illuminates a New and Hopeful Path to a Cure* (CreateSpace Independent Publishing Platform, 2014), 147–48.

7   Gonzalez, Nicholas James, and Isaacs, Linda Lee, "Evaluation of Pancreatic Proteolytic Enzyme Treatment of Adenocarcinoma of the Pancreas, With Nutrition and Detoxification Support," *Nutrition and Cancer* 1999;33(2):117–24. http://www.dr-gonzalez.com/pilot_study_abstract.htm.

8   Saruc, M., et al., "Pancreatic Enzyme Extract Improves Survival in Murine Pancreatic Cancer," *Pancreas*, 2004 May;28(4):401—12. http://www.dr-gonzalez.com/mice04.htm.

9   Gonzalez, Nicholas, and Isaacs, Linda, "The Gonzalez Therapy and Cancer: A Collection of Case Reports," *Alternative Therapies in Health and Medicine*, 2007 Jan/Feb;13(1):46–55. http://www.alternative-therapies.com/at/web_pdfs/gonzalez1.pdf.

10   Gonzalez, Nicholas, "Enzyme Therapy and Cancer," Dr-Gonzalez.com. http://www.dr-gonzalez.com/history_of_treatment.htm.

11   "The Gerson Therapy," The Gerson Institute, 2011. http://gerson.org/gerpress/the-gerson-therapy/.

12   "Issels Immunotherapy—Advanced Immuno-Oncology Treatment of Cancers," Issels Immuno-Oncology. http://www.issels.com/newissels/treatment-summary/

13   "Macrobiotic diet," Cancer Research U.K. http://www.cancerresearchuk.org/about-cancer/cancers-in-general/treatment/complementary-alternative/therapies/macrobiotic-diet.

14   "Contreras Alternative Cancer Treatment (C-ACT)," Oasis of Hope Hospital. http://www.oasisofhope.com/cancer-treatments/contreras-alternative-cancer-treatment-c-act/.

15   Quirós, Pedro, et al., "New roles for mitochondrial proteases in health, ageing and disease," *Nature Reviews Molecular Cell Biology*, 2015 May;16:345–59. http://www.nature.com/nrm/journal/v16/n6/abs/nrm3984.html.

16   "Systemic, Proteolytic Enzymes," The Best Proteolytic Enzymes Formula, Baseline of Health Foundation, 2014. http://jonbarron.org/article/proteolytic-enzyme-formula.

17   Poff, Angela, et al., "The Ketogenic Diet and Hyperbaric Oxygen Therapy Prolong Survival in Mice with Systemic Metastatic Cancer," *PLOS One*, 2013;8(6):e65522. http://journals.plos.org/plosone/article?id=10.1371/journal.pone.0065522

18   Berkhan, Martin, Leangains.com. http://www.leangains.com.

19   Marziali, Carl, "Fasting weakens cancer in mice," *USC News*, February 8, 2012. https://news.usc.edu/29428/fasting-weakens-cancer-in-mice/.

20   Christofferson, Travis, *Tripping Over the Truth: The Return of the Metabolic Theory of Cancer Illuminates a New and Hopeful Path to a Cure* (CreateSpace Independent Publishing Platform, 2014), 204.

INDEX

oleic acid as protection against, 193–194
ozone therapy, 227
predisposition by bisphenol-A, 115
RIGVIR treatment, 242
SP-Activate treatment for, 199–201
thymidine kinase test, 131–132
Breast Cancer Action (BCAction), 95
Breast Cancer Awareness Month, 125
Breast Cancer Conqueror protocol, 140
Bristol-Myers Squibb, 96
Brown, Jerry, 70
Brusch, Charles (Dr.), 162
Bucey, Jared, 80–81, 183–185
Buckthorn (*Rhamnus frangula*), 166, 169
Burdock root (*Arctium lappa*), 38, 163, 166, 183
Burke, James, 40–41
Burzynski, Stanislaw (Dr.), 80
Buttar, Rashid (Dr.), 178–179
Buttram, Harold E., 72

Cade, Helen ("Mama Helen"), 160–161
Cagan, Michele, 130
Caisse, Rene, 161–162
Calbom, Cherie ("The Juice Lady"), 191
California Chiropractic Association, 70
Callender, Cassandra, 79–80
Cameron, Ewan (Dr.), 231–232
Canada, cancer treatment in, 98, 161–162
Cancer
  absence in ancient civilizations, 92–93
  as death sentence, xiii, xix
  as genetic disease, 101–102
  as man-made disease, 93
  as metabolic disease, 259–260
  as normal body reaction, 120–121
  case against chemo, 74–78
  causes of, 87–92, 101–102
  diagnosis/deaths, estimates, xvii, 93–95
  effectiveness of alternative treatments, xviii
  integrative treatment approach, xix, 30–31, 138–141, 271, 279
  overcoming ignorance about, 85–86
  treatment costs, 95–99

Cancer (journal), 42
Cancer, Causes & Control (journal), 115
Cancer and Clinical Oncology (journal), 131–132
Cancer and Vitamin C (Pauling & Cameron), 232
Cancer prevention
  avoiding toxins, 145–153
  God-like power of FDA over, 67–68
  holistic healing and, 3
  holistic lifestyle and, 137–139, 159–160, 194, 279
  immune system, importance, 18
  metabolic therapy, 265–271
  nutrition and role of enzymes, 154–155
  physical/aerobic exercise, 141–144
  proteolytic enzymes, 261–265, 272–274
  role of autophagy, 257–261
  screening/early detection, 104–105, 122–126
  spiritual and emotional grounding, 139–141
  weight training, 144–145
The Cancer Prevention Book (Daniel), 138–139
Cancer remediation, 191
  cancer-fighting foods, 188–194
  cannabis (hemp), 169–175
  detox/cleansing protocols, 175–185
  Essiac tea, 160–165
  Gerson therapy, 185–188, 267–268
  Hoxsey Tonic, 165–169
  lifestyle changes and, 159–160
Cancer screening
  belief that more is better, 120–121, 125–126
  biomarkers, 126, 129, 132
  early detection risks/benefits, 104–105, 119–120, 122–126, 131, 134
  mammograms, dangers of, 122–124
  PSA test, dangers of, 124–125
  safer alternatives, 126–135
Cancer: Step Outside the Box (Bollinger), 87, 144
Candida. *See* Yeast, fungi, and mold
Cannabis (hemp), 169–175, 194, 254
Carcinogenesis, 254

Essiac tea, 160–165, 169, 175, 183, 194
Essential oils
    anticancer properties, 250–255
    antioxidant properties, 248, 252
    breast cancer treatment, 252–253
    effects on immune system, 248
    response of viruses, 248–250, 256
    role in plants, 248–249
Eucalyptus, 249
Excitotoxins (aspartame, MSG), 147–149
Excitotoxins: The Taste That Kills
    (Blaylock), 148
Experimental medicine, 16–17
Experimental Neurobiology (journal), 258
Expert Review of Molecular Diagnostics, 132

Faith. *See* God/faith in God
Farr, Charles H. (Dr.), 222, 228–229
Fasting, 275–276
Fats and hydrogenated oils. *See also*
    Omega-3/-6 fats, 145–146, 186, 188–189, 231, 267, 274
Fell, J. W. (Dr.), 39
Fenn, Alan J. (Dr.), 213
Fermentation/fermentation process
    cancer-fighting foods, 192–193
    cellular respiration of sugars, 91, 147
    hiding MSG in foods, 148
    pasteurization stops, 12–14
    role of bacteria, 15
Fermented foods
    cancer-fighting foods, 189–193
    natural health cure, xiv
    probiotics, 237
    use in holistic nutrition, 214, 269
Fibrosarcoma, 129
Fibromyalgia, 149, 171
First Amendment (U.S. Constitution), 74
Fishbein, Morris (Dr.), 42
Fisher, Howard (Dr.), 209
Fitzgerald, Benedict, 41
Fitzgerald Report, 41–45
Flexner, Abraham, 21, 24–26
Flexner, Simon, 25–26
Flexner Report. *See* Medical education
"Flexner Report—100 Years Later"
    (Duffy), 27

Fluoride, linkage to cancer, 114–115, 152–153
Food, Drug, and Cosmetic Act of 1938, 57
Food and Drug Administration (FDA), 108–109
    aspartame approval, 149
    closing the Hoxsey Clinics, 40–42
    creation of, 57
    drug development costs, 65–66
    pharmaceutical approval, 68
    restricting imported drugs, 98–99
    safety testing of GMOs, 109–110
    support of "Big Pharma," 55
    suppressing natural therapies, 44, 67–68, 79–80, 262
    virotherapy approval, 239–240
Formaldehyde, 111–112, 116, 149
Frankfurter, Felix, 54
Freud, Sigmund, 51, 54
Functional medicine. *See* Integrative medicine
Fungi. *See* Yeast, fungi, and mold

Gagarin, Yuri, 205
Gallbladder cleanse, 182
Gastrointestinal disorders, 109–110, 132, 149–150, 164, 215–217, 224
GcMAF (group specific component macrophage activating factor), 132–133
The GcMAF Book 2.0 (Smith), 128, 132–133
Genesis 1:29–30, 187
Genetically modified organisms (GMOs), 108, 109–110, 114, 149–150, 242
Genetics/genetic damage
    bisphenol-A (BPA), 115–116
    causes of cancer?, 101–102, 259–260
    cellular health and, 152–153, 276
    fluoride mutagenicity, 114–115
Germ theory
    defined, 8
    origins/development, 8–9
    Pasteur and, 12–13, 16–18
    research by Béchamp and Bernard, 14–16
German model of medicine, 27–28, 32–33

Gerson, Max (Dr.), xiv, 185
Gerson Clinic (Tijuana, Mex.), 186
Gerson Therapy, 185–188, 267–268
Getzendanner, Susan, 47
Ghost articles, 58–59
Gleevac (leukemia drug), 98
Gliomas (tumor), 114
Glum, Gary (Dr.), 162
Glutathione reductase (GR), 253
Glyphosate (Roundup herbicide),
107–109
God/faith in God, role in healing, xv
Goebbels, Joseph, 53
Gonzalez, Nicholas (Dr.), 261–267,
270–271
Good, Robert, 263
Goodman, Ira (Dr.), 260
Gout, 226
Great Medical Hoax, 23–27, 44, 70
Gregg, David (Dr.), 89–90
Group, Edward F., III (Dr.), 177
Gunderman, Richard, 53, 54
Gunpoint medicine, 78–81

Hammack, Trina, 201–203
Harris, Malcolm (Dr.), 40
Hartwell, Jonathan, 39
HCA (heterocyclic amines), 117
hCG Urine Immunoassay, 129
Health Progress (journal), 140
Health Reformer (journal), 225–226
Health-defining behavior, 138
Heart disease, 95, 138, 145–147, 222
Heavy metals, 111, 113, 123, 178–179,
267
Hepatitis B, 71, 72–73
The Herb Quarterly (journal), 39
Herbal medicine
Asclepiadean approach, 6
before/after Flexner Report, 22–23,
29, 32
elimination of Hoxsey Clinics,
37–41
switch to drugs and surgery, 49–50
Herbal remedies
cannabis (hemp), 169–175, 194, 254
Essiac tea, 160–165, 169, 175, 183,
194
Hoxsey tonic, 34–35, 37–42,
165–169, 183, 194

treatment with, 159–160
Herbicides. *See* Pesticides
Herd immunity, 70
Herlihy, Brian Patrick, 73
Herpes, 103, 239, 242
Hertel, Hans (Dr.), 151
High-dose vitamin C injections, 231–
234, 236
High-energy water, 209–212
High-radio-frequency (RF) generators,
208–209
High-resolution blood analysis, 123
High-resolution blood analysis [HRB]
(alternative screening), 134–135
Hilu, Raymond (Dr.), 122, 134–135
Hippocrates of Kos, 3–9
Hippocratic Oath, 6, 8
HIV (human immunodeficiency virus)
bio-oxidative therapies, 222
burdock root benefits, 163
growth in absence of GcMAF, 133
hydrogen peroxide therapy, 230
ozone therapy, 224
THC benefits, 171–172
Hodgkin lymphoma, 79–81, 212
Holistic medicine, from Asclepiades,
3–7
Holman, Reginald (Dr.), 229
Homeopathy, 22, 29, 32, 268, 277
Hope4Cancer Institute (Mex.), 197–
204, 214, 217, 222, 275–276
Hopkins Circle, 25
Hosea 4:6, xviii–xix
Hoxsey, Harry, 37–38, 40
Hoxsey, John, 37–38
Hoxsey Tonic
challenging the new medical system,
34–35
eliminated as alternate treatment,
37–42
preparation and use, 165–169, 194
side effects/health risks, 169
use as cleansing tonic, 183
Huish, Allison, 255
Human papillomavirus (HPV), 103
"Humors," Hippocratic theory of, 5–6,
8
Hunsaker, Jonathan, 315
Hydrogen peroxide therapy, 228–231
Hyperacute encephalitis, 72

Plamer, Daniel David ("D. D."), 45
Plants Used Against Cancer (Hartwell), 38–39
Plastics/bisphenol-A, 111, 115–116, 151, 253
PLOS ONE (journal), 76
Pneumonia, 189, 226
Politics, suppression of alternatives, xviii–xix
Pollutants. *See* Environmental contamination
Potassium iodide, 38, 165
Potassium levels/supplements, 169, 186, 206, 267
Precepts (Asclepiades), 6
President's Cancer Panel, 105, 108–109
"The Prime Cause and Prevention of Cancer" (Warburg), 91
Pritchett, Henry S., 26, 29
Probiotics. *See also* Bacteria
  beneficial effects, 18, 237, 256
  component in curing cancer, xiv, 250
  immune stimulation therapy, 270
  raw milk as source of, 153
  supplementing a colon cleanse, 180
Proceedings of the International Conference on Bio-Oxidative Medicine, 228
Proceedings of the National Academy of Sciences, 147
Processed meats, 117
Propaganda (Bernays), 52
Prostate cancer
  diagnosis/deaths estimates, 94–95
  enzyme therapy, 264
  heat therapy, 217
  oleic acid as protection against, 193–194
  pesticide exposure, 108
  PSA test/prostate biopsy, 120, 124–125
  RIGVIR treatment, 242
  SP-Activate treatment for, 199–201
Proteolytic enzyme therapy, 261–265, 272–274
PSA test
  benefits/risks, 119–120
  dangers of, 124–125
  pros/cons of screening, 125–126

screening alternatives, 126–128
Psychological manipulation, 54
Psychoneuroimmunology (PNI), 139
PubMed (online search engine), xvii
Puig, Oscar, 276
Pulsed electromagnetic fields, 204–207, 218
Pulsed intravenous vitamin C, 233–234
PVC (polyvinyl chloride), 111, 116, 151
Pyrethrum (pesticide), 106–107
Pythagoream theorem, 4–6

Quackery
  competing alternatives as, 29–32
  labeling by the AMA, 40–42, 56
  natural medicines and herbs as, 49–50, 66
"The Quack Who Cured Cancer" (Burke), 41
The Quest for the Cures (Bell), 23
Quillin, Patrick (Dr.), 63–64, 170

Rabies, 13, 242
Radiation
  alternative screening, 126–135
  alternative treatments, 160–161, 171, 175, 195, 279
  as cause of cancer, 42, 62, 89, 113–114, 123–126, 178
  coercion to use, 67, 78–79
  as "conventional option," xix, 51, 55, 120
  effectiveness/side effects, 39, 43, 86, 93, 119–120, 221, 271
  promotion as cancer cure, 70
Radio frequencies (RF). *See* Electromagnetic devices/frequencies
Radiological Society of North America, 123
Rainbow Diet, 153
Refined sugar/high-fructose corn syrup, 146–147, 150, 153
Resistance
  cancer cells, 75–76
  insulin, 153, 275–276
  pesticides, 107–108
Resperin's Original Caisse Formula Tea, 162
Rife, Royal Raymond (Dr.), 35–37, 45, 208

Riordan, Hugh (Dr.), 232
R-KD (Restricted Ketogenic Diet),
274–275
Rockefeller Foundation, 23–35, 56
Rockefeller Institute, 26
Roosevelt, Franklin D., 54, 57

Salk polio vaccine, 113
Sarcoma, 113, 115, 129, 246
Schönbein, Christian Friedrich, 223
Schulze, Richard (Dr.), 183
Sea kelp (*Laminariales*), 38
Seeger, Paul Gerhardt, 90, 91–92
"Seven toxicities," 178–179
Seyfried, Thomas, 260, 275–276
Shaken baby syndrome (SBS), 72–73
Sherman Antitrust Act of 1890, 47
Simpson, Rick, 174
Sircus, Mark (Dr.), 147
Skin cancer, 95–96, 108, 129
Sleep/circadian rhythm, 143, 153, 172,
206
Smallpox, 10–11, 13
Smirnov, Igor (Dr.), 209
Smith, Jeffrey M., 110, 150
Smith, Tim (Dr.), 128, 132–133
Smith, Trevor and Carol, 175
Sokolova, Zoya, 246–247
Sound (sonodynamic) therapy, 197–
204, 218
SP-Activate (sensitizing agent), 199–201
Spiritual health, cancer prevention and,
137–141, 159, 178, 197, 271
Spontaneous generation, 14–19
Starvation mode (intermittent fasting),
276
Stem cell therapy, 259, 268–269
Stem cells, turning cancer into, 75–76,
89, 240
Stephenson, Michael, 217
Stomach cancer
dealing with diagnosis of, xvii
eating processed meats, 117
Essiac tea, 161
maitake mushroom extract, 191
natural health cure, xiii–xiv
RIGVIR therapy, 247
Sudden infant death syndrome (SIDS), 72
Sun
ancient beliefs of healing, 196

healing properties, 200, 218, 235
protection from sunburn, 196, 218
Sweating, detoxification by, 141–142
Symptoms
managing with drugs, 9
origin of term, 5

Tamoxifen (drug), 98, 125
Tea tree, 249
Tesla, Nikola, 226
Tetanus, 72–73, 113, 233
THC (tetrahydrocannabinol), 171–175
Thermography, 126–127
Thompson, William (Dr.), 74
Thymidine kinase test, 131–132
Thyroid/thyroid cancer, 95, 115, 151,
165, 186, 267
Titus Aufidius of Sicily, 7
TK1 testing (thymidine kinase test),
131–132
Tobacco (marketing campaign), 53, 55
Tobey, Charles, 41
Trans fats. *See* Fats and hydrogenated
oils
Tribeca Film Festival (New York City),
74
Tripping Over the Truth (Christofferson),
260
The Truth About Cancer: A Global Quest
(Bollinger), 58, 61, 62
Tuberculosis, 13, 185
Tumor necrosis factor, 268
Tumor(s)
alteration of cellular metabolism,
90–91, 275
angiogenesis (blood vessel formation), 90, 249
antineoplaston treatment, 80
as normal body reaction, 87–88,
121–122
chemotherapy delivery, 76
essential oils effects on, 249–250
genetic mutation/variability,
101–102, 260
Hoxsey Tonic properties, 39
immune system failure, 102–104
mutating and spreading cells,
122–124
sugar as fuel for, 147
waste products, 264

Turmeric (curcumin), 189
Turner, Sylvester, 74
T-VEC (talimogene laherparepvec), 239

Ulcerative colitis, 224
Ultraviolet blood irradiation (UBI), 234–236
United Patients Group, 172
Universal prismatic microscope, 36
Unsworth, John, 107
Urbaniak, Eva (Dr.), 166
U.S. Centers for Disease Control and Prevention (CDC), 71, 74, 112
U.S. Constitution, 74
U.S. Preventive Services Task Force, 124

Vaccinations/vaccinology
    "Big Pharma" myths/takeover, 55–59
    derived from chemical weapons, 59–61
    mandatory vs. freedom of choice, 69–74
    opt-out provisions, 69–70
    origins, 9
Vaccine(s). See also Immunity
    development of smallpox, 9–12
    linkage to autism, 68–69, 74, 113
    MBV (mixed bacterial vaccine), 212
    Pasteur's contributions, 9–14
    side effects/health risks, 11, 112–113, 255
    treatment of cancer, 212, 242–243, 268
Vaccinophobia, 73
Van Straten, Arlene, 264–265
Variolation, 11
Vaxxed (film), 74
Venereal disease, 52
Verkerk, Rob (Dr.), 105
Virchow, Rudolph, 17–18
Virotherapeutics
    benefits from "friendly" viruses, 237–238
    genetics (enter Big Pharma), 239, 242, 248
    RIGVIR therapy, 239–248, 256
Virus(es)
    as disease vector, 14

control, therapies to, 208, 211, 222–227
detox protocols, 177–178, 180, 182
immune system suppression, 103–105
presence in cancer cells, 35–37
presence in vaccines, 112–113
production of Nagalase, 133
response to essential oils, 248–250, 256
response to herbal remedies, 163
Vitamins and minerals, xviii, 152, 154, 188, 192, 214, 263, 265–267
vitamin B17, 175, 187
vitamin C, 175, 231–234, 236, 270
vitamin D, 64, 102, 175, 189, 196, 218
vitamin K, 270

Wagner-Jauregg, Julius, 213
Wakefield, Andrew (Dr.), 68–69
Walters, Richard, 39
Warburg, Otto, 90–91, 206, 219, 259
Wassell, William (Dr.), 232
Water
    chlorination/organochlorines, 152
    importance of hydration, 153
    MRET therapy, 209–212
    purification with ozone, 227
Watson, James P. (Dr.), 259
Wild indigo root (Baptisia tinctoria), 38
Wilk, Chester, 45–46
Wilk v. AMA (1976), 46–47
Wilson, Woodrow, 52
Wisconsin v. Morikubo (1907), 46
Wolfe, Darrell (Dr.), 31–32
Wolfe, Marcel, 207
Wollams, Chris, 153
Wong, William (Dr.), 151
World Health Organization, xvii, 94, 112, 117, 163
World War I, 52, 61
World War II, 53–54, 60–61, 106
Wright, Jonathan V. (Dr.), 62

X-ray therapy. See Radiation

Yakonvenko, Khrystyna, 244
Yale Journal of Biology and Medicine, 33

ACKNOWLEDGMENTS

I want to acknowledge my wonderful wife, Charlene, who is my "princess" and my best friend. She is my "dream girl" and bride of 20 years, my business partner, and the mother of our four children, Brianna, Bryce, Tabitha, and Charity. She truly is my inspiration, a gift straight from God, the most shining example of His grace in my life and my most passionate encourager. She truly is the "wind beneath my wings." Thank you, Princess, for all that you are, for all that you do, and for our four beautiful children!

My friend Dr. Nicholas Gonzalez was probably the world's foremost expert on cancer, often recommended by other alternative doctors as the "go-to doctor" with the best results for supposedly "terminal" cancers. He loved helping people and sharing his knowledge. Dr. Nick, you are sorely missed!

I also want to acknowledge our "The Truth About Cancer" business partner, Jonathan Hunsaker. Little did we know back in 2014 the impact we would have on the entire world. I can tell you that it's been an awesome ride and this is only the beginning. God definitely connected us and caused our paths to cross. Without your marketing expertise and business acumen, we would never have been able to reach tens of millions of people with the truth about cancer. Thanks, bro! We're changing the world and saving lives! Rock on!

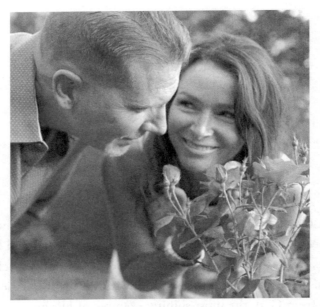

Ty and Charlene Bollinger

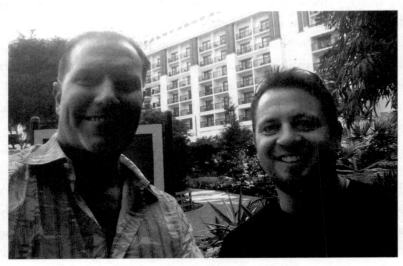

Ty Bollinger and Jonathan Hunsaker

ABOUT THE AUTHOR

Ty Bollinger is a happily married husband and father, Christian, CPA, health freedom advocate, health researcher, former competitive bodybuilder, talk radio host, documentary film producer, and best-selling author. After losing several family members to cancer (including his mother and father), Ty refused to accept the notion that chemotherapy, radiation, and surgery were the most effective treatments available for cancer patients. He began a quest to learn all he possibly could about alternative cancer treatments and the medical industry. What he uncovered was shocking.

In 2006, after almost a decade of cancer research, he published *Cancer—Step Outside the Box* (now in its sixth edition), which has become a bestseller and has been called the "most eye-opening book since *1984*." He went on to author or coauthor several more books on alternative health and the medical industry.

In the spring of 2014, Ty and his wife, Charlene, teamed up with Jonathan Hunsaker, forming The Truth About Cancer, and proceeded to travel across the U.S. and interview the most renowned doctors and scientists about treating cancer naturally. They eventually produced the documentary miniseries (docuseries) entitled *The Quest for The Cures* and *The Quest for The Cures . . . Continues*. This docuseries was viewed by over 2 million people worldwide. In 2015 Ty traveled the globe to interview more doctors, scientists, and cancer survivors and produced *The Truth About Cancer: A Global Quest* which aired in October 2015 and April 2016 and has been viewed by over 8 million people worldwide.

Ty and Charlene are co-owners of their multiple health businesses and are working together to change the world. Ty speaks frequently at seminars, expos, conferences, and churches; is a regular guest on multiple radio shows; and writes for numerous magazines and websites. He has appeared many times on FOX News, and he cohosts a weekly radio show (along with Robert Scott Bell) called *Outside the Box Wednesdays*.

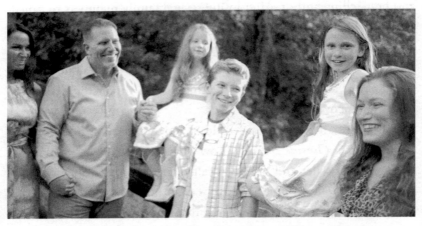

From left to right: Charlene, Ty, Charity, Bryce, Tabitha, and Brianna Bollinger

Hay House Titles of Related Interest

YOU CAN HEAL YOUR LIFE, the movie, starring Louise Hay & Friends
(available as a 1-DVD program and an expanded 2-DVD set)
Watch the trailer at: www.LouiseHayMovie.com

THE SHIFT, the movie,
starring Dr. Wayne W. Dyer
(available as a 1-DVD program and an expanded 2-DVD set)
Watch the trailer at: www.DyerMovie.com

***

THE BONE BROTH SECRET: A Culinary Adventure in Health, Beauty, and Longevity, by Louise Hay and Heather Dane

CULTURED FOOD FOR HEALTH: A Guide to Healing Yourself with Probiotic Foods, by Donna Schwenk

KALE AND COFFEE: A Renegade's Guide to Health, Happiness, and Longevity, by Kevin Gianni

REAL FOOD REVOLUTION: Healthy Eating, Green Groceries, and the Return of the American Family Farm, by Congressman Tim Ryan

All of the above are available at www.hayhouse.co.uk

***

NOTES

NOTES

NOTES

NOTES

HAY HOUSE

Look within

Join the conversation about latest products,
events, exclusive offers and more.

f Hay House UK

🐦 @HayHouseUK

📷 @hayhouseuk

❤️ healyourlife.com

We'd love to hear from you!